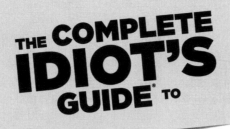

THE **COMPLETE IDIOT'S GUIDE** TO

Triathlon Training

D0565356

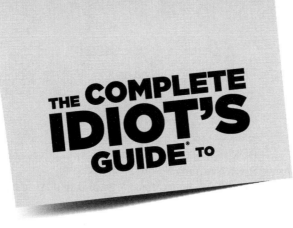

THE COMPLETE IDIOT'S GUIDE® TO

Triathlon Training

by Colin Barr and Steve Katai

ALPHA

A member of Penguin Group (USA) Inc.

ALPHA BOOKS

Published by the Penguin Group

Published by the Penguin Group

Penguin Group (USA) Inc., 375 Hudson Street, New York, New York 10014, USA

Penguin Group (Canada), 90 Eglinton Avenue East, Suite 700, Toronto, Ontario M4P 2Y3, Canada (a division of Pearson Penguin Canada Inc.)

Penguin Books Ltd., 80 Strand, London WC2R 0RL, England

Penguin Ireland, 25 St. Stephen's Green, Dublin 2, Ireland (a division of Penguin Books Ltd.)

Penguin Group (Australia), 250 Camberwell Road, Camberwell, Victoria 3124, Australia (a division of Pearson Australia Group Pty. Ltd.)

Penguin Books India Pvt. Ltd., 11 Community Centre, Panchsheel Park, New Delhi—110 017, India

Penguin Group (NZ), 67 Apollo Drive, Rosedale, North Shore, Auckland 1311, New Zealand (a division of Pearson New Zealand Ltd.)

Penguin Books (South Africa) (Pty.) Ltd., 24 Sturdee Avenue, Rosebank, Johannesburg 2196, South Africa

Penguin Books Ltd., Registered Offices: 80 Strand, London WC2R 0RL, England

Copyright © 2007 by TRI Guys

All rights reserved. No part of this book shall be reproduced, stored in a retrieval system, or transmitted by any means, electronic, mechanical, photocopying, recording, or otherwise, without written permission from the publisher. No patent liability is assumed with respect to the use of the information contained herein. Although every precaution has been taken in the preparation of this book, the publisher and authors assume no responsibility for errors or omissions. Neither is any liability assumed for damages resulting from the use of information contained herein. For information, address Alpha Books, 800 East 96th Street, Indianapolis, IN 46240.

THE COMPLETE IDIOT'S GUIDE TO and Design are registered trademarks of Penguin Group (USA) Inc.

International Standard Book Number: 978-1-59257-580-0
Library of Congress Catalog Card Number: 2006936692

13   12   11   9   8   7

Interpretation of the printing code: The rightmost number of the first series of numbers is the year of the book's printing; the rightmost number of the second series of numbers is the number of the book's printing. For example, a printing code of 07-1 shows that the first printing occurred in 2007.

Printed in the United States of America

Note: This publication contains the opinions and ideas of its authors. It is intended to provide helpful and informative material on the subject matter covered. It is sold with the understanding that the authors and publisher are not engaged in rendering professional services in the book. If the reader requires personal assistance or advice, a competent professional should be consulted.

The authors and publisher specifically disclaim any responsibility for any liability, loss, or risk, personal or otherwise, which is incurred as a consequence, directly or indirectly, of the use and application of any of the contents of this book.

Most Alpha books are available at special quantity discounts for bulk purchases for sales promotions, premiums, fund-raising, or educational use. Special books, or book excerpts, can also be created to fit specific needs.

For details, write: Special Markets, Alpha Books, 375 Hudson Street, New York, NY 10014.

Publisher: *Marie Butler-Knight*
Editorial Director: *Mike Sanders*
Managing Editor: *Billy Fields*
Senior Acquisitions Editor: *Paul Dinas*
Senior Development Editor: *Christy Wagner*
Production Editor: *Megan Douglass*
Copy Editor: *Emily Garner*

Cartoonist: *Shannon Wheeler*
Cover Designer: *Kurt Owens*
Book Designer: *Trina Wurst*
Indexer: *Brad Herriman*
Layout: *Brian Massey*
Proofreader: *Aaron Black*

Contents at a Glance

Contents

Introduction

You're cordially invited to come with us on a journey into the sport of triathlon. This is a journey that might change your life for the better, as it has ours, and as it has for thousands of people across the world. If you're curious about triathlon or looking for an adventure, keep reading. In these pages, you will learn. You will be inspired. You will succeed. Be prepared to challenge yourself and show your desire to achieve.

At this point, you might not even be sure what a triathlon is. The standard triathlon consists of swimming, biking, and running, in that order. Generally, the swim is the shortest segment of the race and the bike the longest. Between each of the sports is a period called transition, where athletes enter a designated area to leave equipment and clothing they no longer need and pick up equipment and clothing they need going forward. That's it in a nutshell.

If you want to start doing triathlons for fun, fitness, weight loss, or any other reason, you'll benefit from this book. For those of you who have already started down the TRI path, we help you get to the next level. Our goal is to be your partners on a successful and rewarding triathlon journey.

But be warned: *This sport may become an addiction. Participation in triathlon may cause feelings of improved self-confidence, an increased sense of accomplishment, and overall good health. Prolonged use may cause endorphin highs to course through your veins and make you feel generally better about life.*

Many people we know started out triathlon with the mind-set: *I'll try this once.* But like a famous potato chip ad, you can't do just one. These "just one" folks are still *totally* hooked on triathlon. They appear more fit, feel healthier, and enjoy treating their bodies right. They even enjoy early morning runs. Be careful … this could happen to you!

How did you even start thinking about going down this path? Perhaps you were stopped in your car in traffic so some competing triathletes could cross the road and you wondered, *What's all that about?* Maybe a friend started doing triathlons and you thought, *I should give that a try.* Maybe you've seen the Hawaii Ironman on TV and thought, *That is amazing!* You might have done one or two triathlons but felt like you needed a little more organization or motivation in your training. No matter your reason, here you are with this road map in front of you.

There are no physical prerequisites for you to start getting into this great sport. You don't have to know how to swim, ride a bike, or run—yet. Nobody is born with these skills; they are learned. You will pick up and/or improve in any area you're lacking. If you're already proficient at any of these three skills, you're ahead of the game. We help you feel confident in all three sports and help you put them together as one.

Maybe you've already done a few triathlons and you're looking to improve your experience/results. We'll get you there. The training programs in this book, along with the insightful commentary and observations, will take your game to the next level.

Everyone has a reason why they *can't* get into triathlon. If we had a dollar for every time we heard, "I'd love to do a triathlon but I can't because I don't have time" or "… because I can't swim that well" or "… because I don't like running," we'd be rich. There's always a reason why a person *can't* do something. You simply need to decide that you *will* do it and then *get it done!*

We have seen athletes without legs use special equipment to complete triathlons of all lengths. Mothers with several children and a full-time job cross the finish line at every triathlon. Men and women in their 70s and 80s compete in TRI every year. We've seen a hero carry his paralyzed son across every mile of a 140.6-mile triathlon. If your reasons for "can't" are not quite as powerful, we hope you decide right now to commit yourself to this journey of a lifetime.

Triathlon is great for people of all sizes and shapes. Swimming and biking are great ways to help you get started in a no-impact or low-impact way. If you are physically challenged in any way, several equipment options are available that can help you in this journey. If there's a will, there's a way!

The beauty of this sport is that everyone involved wants you to succeed. They will pick you up when you're down and when you don't think you could make it another step. They will give you encouragement even while you're passing them on the course.

The only real requirements for this sport are passion, desire, and attitude. Do you have what it takes? We know you do. Now you must decide for yourself. The voyage will require some dedication from you; we'll supply the inspiration, explanation, and motivation. Let's get it started.

How to Use This Book

So what's in this book?

In **Part 1, "Just TRI It,"** we introduce you to triathlon and explain what you need to join the movement that's sweeping the nation.

In **Part 2, "You Got Skills, and They're Multiplyin',"** we cover the components of triathlon: swimming, biking, running, and transition, and give you tips on improving your skills in all four areas.

Part 3, "Beyond the Four Disciplines of Triathlon," is where we cover the *other* four parts of triathlon: nutrition, weight training, stretching, and getting enough rest. Even the most elite athletes sometimes forget this important part of the triathlon equation.

In **Part 4, "Realizing Your Dream,"** we bring you up to the big day—race day!—and share with you what that day will be like. After reading through this book, when you wake up on race day, you will be ready.

In the back of the book, we've included a glossary of TRI terms and an appendix of suggested resources so you can continue your quest for more information on triathlon.

Extras

Throughout the text you'll see some boxed asides:

def•i•ni•tion

These boxes offer definitions for terms that help you better understand the triathlon jargon.

Gravel Ahead

You'll want to heed these warnings to avoid potential pitfalls.

Training Tips

Check out these boxes for helpful tips to make training and racing more efficient and enjoyable.

Coaches' Corner

Here you'll find commentary and anecdotes from us, Colin and Steve, as well as some coach-worthy advice.

Acknowledgments

We wouldn't be here if it wasn't for the influence of others. We wanted to both acknowledge and thank some of those people for their involvement and support (in no special order):

Thanks to Paul Dinas, our acquisitions editor, for seeing value in us and our vision for this book project. And thanks to the editors and production staff at Alpha. We appreciate your direction, coaching, and efforts.

A big thank you goes out to Multisports.com: Huddle, Roch, Newby, Heather, and Duke. Your expert triathlon coaching, advice, and friendship have made all the difference.

We cannot say enough about our TRI mentor, Bob Babbitt. Bob is a special man who has contributed so much to the sport. Thank you, Cleatus, for all you do, have done, and just for being you.

We also want to acknowledge a couple of our original TRI mentors, with whom we spent countless hours on the bike: Paul Healing (Steve) and Donna Phelan (Colin). Thank you for taking your time to make sure we were prepared for the challenge of a lifetime.

We want to thank Lois Schwartz, for contributing most of the race photos found in the book. Your brilliant work in photography and talent for capturing action over the years is appreciated and is a great addition to the book.

Thank you, Todd Schoelen, for shooting the stretching photos and the use of your gym (CORE).

A tip of the hat to Peter Baiamonte for permission to use your exercise photos that appear in Chapter 10.

Thanks to Meghan Duffy and Eric Gibson for your graphic design support. And to Krysia Kij for supporting us on our proposal.

From Steve: thanks to my wife, Noelle. You have always been there supporting me in all my life's pursuits. You are a source of light, love, and happiness. My family: Mom, Dad, Melissa, Maria, Josh, and all my relatives. You gave me life and perpetual life coaching. My friends: thanks for the unconditional camaraderie and support. Colin: you have been an incredible partner (coauthor). I've thoroughly enjoyed spending the long hours working with you on our book project. It's been a rewarding journey to say the least.

From Colin: thanks to my beautiful girlfriend, Bonnie, who puts up with all my antics and insanity and stands by me through it all. I'm so lucky to have found you. To my parents, Larry and Sherry, and my sister, Eileen, for their undying love and support in all my endeavors. To Sara, who helped in the initial proposal of this project and gave encouragement along the way (as you always do). To the rest of my family and friends: thank you for always being patient with me and trying to keep track of my latest exciting adventures. Katai: it's truly been a gratifying process, and I'm glad you were the one to work through it with me (thank goodness for free mobile-to-mobile minutes!).

Special Thanks to Unilever (d.b.a. Degree)

Both of us owe our TRI beginning to the makers of Degree Antiperspirant. If the "Degree Everyman Ironman" Program did not exist, neither of us would be on this path. It was much more than just a contest. It has changed our lives forever and given us the opportunity to pursue our dreams. Many agencies contributed to the DEIM program, but to thank just a few: Weber Shandwick, Active, and 141 Worldwide. We are forever grateful for what you have done.

Trademarks

All terms mentioned in this book that are known to be or are suspected of being trademarks or service marks have been appropriately capitalized. Alpha Books and Penguin Group (USA) Inc. cannot attest to the accuracy of this information. Use of a term in this book should not be regarded as affecting the validity of any trademark or service mark.

Part 1

Just TRI It

Triathlon fever is sweeping the nation. Every year, the number of participants in the sport is growing exponentially, and it's even being featured on prime-time sitcoms. TRI popularity is growing for many reasons, not least of which is the ease of getting involved. As long as you have a pair of running shoes, a swimsuit, and access to a bike, you can take up this sport.

If you like to challenge yourself and have the desire to achieve in the triathlon world, this book is for you. Don't be overwhelmed by any challenge in the world of triathlons—anything is possible if you put your mind to it. If you want to start taking part in triathlons for fun, fitness, weight loss, or any other reason, you have come to the right place. For those of you who have already started down the TRI path, we help you get to the next level.

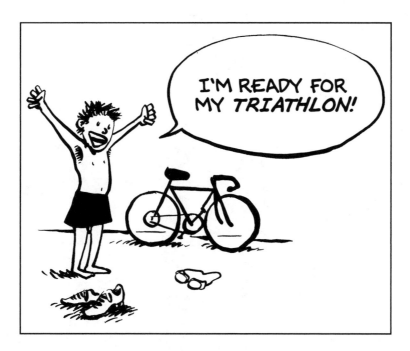

Chapter 1

Why in the World Would a Person Do One of These?

In This Chapter

- ♦ Understanding the roots of the triathlon and how it's evolving
- ♦ Looking at the benefits of training and racing
- ♦ Finding other dimensions within the sport
- ♦ Learning to be comfortable in your own skin

Why conquer a triathlon (TRI)? Answers to that question vary as much as individual personalities do. Some participants like that triathlon offers a new way to push their mind and body. Others enjoy the camaraderie offered by races and local TRI clubs. Others see it as a great way to get fit and lose some weight. And a select few men just want an excuse to shave their legs! Whatever your reason, the TRI world will welcome you with open arms and complete encouragement.

The New Challenge in Town

The public's perception of the triathlon is changing. Steve once saw a comedy routine with a segment on triathletes. The comedian was talking about this rare and crazy breed of athletes who swim around some buoys, then get on their bikes and ride for miles, and finish with a running competition. She was drawing a strong contrast between herself, or "normal" folk, and these "freaks of nature."

It was a funny segment, but the reality is a little different. The old mind-set of triathletes being gluttons for punishment is being replaced with thoughts such as *I can see myself doing that!* We are all lucky to be in on the early stages of this growing sport, and we're going to have a blast riding the wave!

A Unique Sport

More than the all-welcoming attitude or the ease with which you can get involved with TRI, its attraction is its inherent self-challenging framework and the way it impacts those involved. Many individual sports exist—tennis, golf, gymnastics, billiards, etc. Each of these has its own qualities, but none have the same ability to manifest individual evolution and change like TRI.

> **Coaches' Corner**
>
> When you push yourself, you're forced to remove barriers and discover the person you become when you give everything you have. This is a form of personal evolution.

TRI has a magical way of galvanizing growth. When we show up at the starting line, we bring what makes us up— age, weight, fitness level, personality, and attitude. When we cross the finish line, something has inevitably shifted. There's a new sense of self that's created from TRI and the challenges within it.

A Brief History

The first triathlon on record was held in San Diego (Mission Bay), California, in 1974. Forty-six participants, both males and females, took part in a 6-mile run, a 5-mile bike, and a 500-meter swim.

John Collins, one of the athletes who raced that day, helped take the sport to the next level. He took the triathlon concept to Hawaii and in 1978, combined three of Oahu's previously established endurance events—the Waikiki Rough Water Swim, the Around-Oahu Bike Ride, and the Honolulu Marathon—into one, 140.6-mile race: the Ironman.

When triathlon started, only a few brave souls took up the new challenge in town.

(Photo by Lois Schwartz)

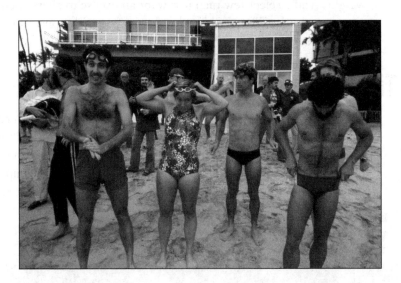

ABC's *Wide World of Sports* televised the event 2 years later. People across the globe were inspired and overwhelmed with emotion as they watched the Ironman athletes truly put their bodies to the ultimate challenge. We were inspired, and that's what initially drove us to the sport. Participation and interest for triathlons of all distances have grown exponentially since the sport's birth. The following table provides a snapshot of some other triathlon milestones.

Triathlon Milestones	
1974	The San Diego Track Club Newsletter advertised its new race with a headline reading "Run, Cycle, Swim—Triathlon set for 25th of September," using the word *triathlon* for the first time in the modern sense.
1978	Fifteen men started the first Iron Man: twelve finished. Gordon Haller became the first Iron Man champion, winning the race in 11 hours, 46 minutes, 58 seconds.
1982	Second-place finisher Julie Moss's unforgettable crawl to the Ironman finish line shown on ABC's *Wide World of Sports* inspired many to take up triathlon. The Torrey Pines Triathlon, won by Dave Scott, was both the first United States Triathlon Series event and the first triathlon to offer prize money.
1993	Actor Tom Cruise completed an 18-mile bicycle leg of the Malibu triathlon as part of a relay team. Other celebrities participating in the sport in subsequent years have included Robin Williams, Jim Carrey, Will Farrell, Jennifer Garner, Alexandra Paul, Alanis Morrisette, Felicity Huffman, William H. Macy, and David Duchovny.
2000	Triathlon debuted as an Olympic sport in Sydney, Australia.
2003	Ironman celebrated its twenty-fifth anniversary in Kona, Hawaii.
2004	Triathlon made its second Olympic appearance in Athens, Greece.

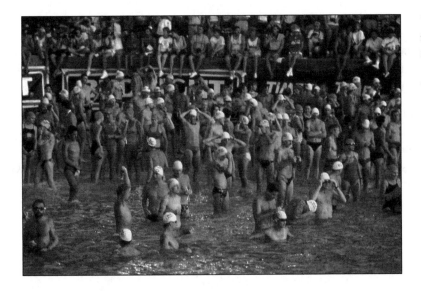

Triathlon has grown exponentially in popularity since its meager beginnings.

(Photo by Lois Schwartz)

True Accomplishment in a World of Immediate Gratification

We live in times of instant messaging, e-mails, direct-connect cell phones, and fast food. With everything seemingly at our fingertips, it becomes very easy to forget about true gratification and expect everything *now*. We seem to have forgotten that the harder we work to reach a goal, the sweeter it is once it's obtained.

TRI provides us the opportunity to set personal goals and work at achieving them. It forces us to put some structure in our lives and strive for greatness.

Enjoying the Journey

The greatest thing about triathlon is, put simply: it can be a lot of fun. It doesn't matter if you're in it for recreation, fitness, or even some friendly competition. We know a lot of tri-athletes with many different goals, but all share a common denominator—passion for the sport. Each workout is an opportunity to get faster, stronger, and leaner. You will become a grander version of yourself: the journey is the reward.

Those who compete in TRI may find it easy to focus on the end result—race day. Although it's good to leverage the finish line for inspiration, remember that TRI is made up of much more than just this one important aspect. Many dimensions go into creating the "mojo" of the sport. During the experience, pay attention to all the parts that make up the sum: individual workouts, friendships, exploring new places, reward foods, the great outdoors, self-improvements. Every day is special.

> **Coaches' Corner**
>
> Steve's favorite self-coined phrase is, "It's a lifestyle: train like there is no finish line."

Playing Full Out

For many of us, the days of gym class and summer vacation from school go way back. We fondly remember playing tag and dodge ball and doing bunny hops with our bikes. We'd come home sweaty, dirty, and covered with grass stains. Those were the days.

TRI gives us a portal back in time. We can return to childhood innocence and simply enjoy the process. Training and racing do not have to be completely serious. Workouts with a purpose are important, but we must always keep things in perspective. Regardless of whether you're a first-time *age grouper* going after *hardware*, or you're a pro going for the *purse*, TRI is essentially about leading a healthy and happy lifestyle—an opportunity to play full out!

def·i·ni·tion

An **age grouper** is any nonprofessional triathlete who competes in triathlon races. Age groupers can compete for **hardware,** which is any award, such as medals or trophies, usually given out to the top finishers per age group. For example, Steve would fall in the M30–34 division. He would be competing against other males (M) in the 30- to 34-year-old age range. Pros often compete for a **purse,** which is typically made up of some monetary amount. They do not compete directly with any age groupers.

The Joy of Finishing

There are a few moments in life that really stand out, ones you will never forget: the birth of a child, college graduation, or the purchase of your first house. No matter what your moments are, they stick with you. Typically the moments that stand out are the ones that required the most effort to achieve. The joy of finishing is directly proportional to invested effort.

This is one reason TRI hooks so many first-timers. It's the feeling you get when you cross the finish line. The exact formula is unknown: there's a mix of emotion, intensity, adrenaline, endorphins, sometimes pain, and the magical factor X. This cannot be explained, only felt. If you've been around the sport or triathletes in general, you may hear about "catching the TRI bug." A big part of it stems from this authentic sensation. Once it's in you, you'll want more.

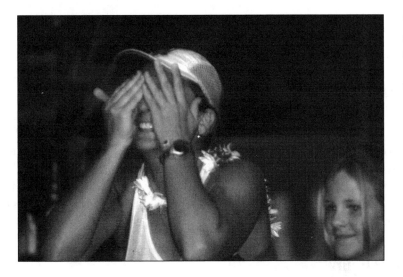

Training has countless benefits, but the joy of finishing is unparalleled.

(Photo by Lois Schwartz)

Breathing Easier and Shedding Some Pounds

TRI is an excellent sport for improving health and fitness. Through training and competition, your body adapts to gradually increased workloads—frequencies, intensities, and durations—and this work enhances your cardio-respiratory function. Your heart, vascular, and respiratory systems all become stronger. In addition, you build more muscle throughout your body and lose fat. The increase in muscle tone contributes to a higher resting metabolic rate. In other words, you burn more calories when you're not even doing anything! The endurance-focus coupled with some of the power and strength components of TRI combine to allow for pure balanced conditioning.

Before Steve got into TRI, he was a gym rat. He worked out with free weights three times a week and focused on max lifts. He was getting strong and thought he was in good shape. However, how he looked in the mirror was deceiving. His cardio endurance was below average, and he had a high resting heart rate. More importantly, his blood pressure and overall health wasn't great.

Within the first 6 months of triathlon training, Steve's resting heart rate fell from 77 beats per minute to 52 beats per minute. He felt better, had more energy, and knew he was on the right track toward longevity and a greater quality of life. He retired his weight belt and never looked back.

Some of the potential health benefits of TRI include the following:

♦ Lower LDL (bad) cholesterol levels in the blood

♦ Higher HDL (good) cholesterol levels in the blood

♦ Reduced chance of strokes and heart attacks

♦ Lower blood pressure

♦ Reduced chance of diabetes

♦ Better overall body composition

Cross-Training: Your Body Will Thank You

Cross-training simply means that you include a variety of exercises or modes in your fitness program. TRI, by nature, employs this principle. A couple of the major benefits are the reduction in boredom and injuries. As a result, the number of people who keep up with their workout regiment increases dramatically. Fitness becomes a lifestyle and no longer a chore. Your mind-set begins to shift from needing to psych yourself up for a workout to not even considering skipping training.

Reducing Your Chance of Injury

One of the unique benefits of this sport is its balanced nature. Swimming, biking, and running are all individual sports that can stand alone. Each one has its own merits. However, over time, each by itself can lead to overuse injuries. For example, a swimmer could experience swimmer's shoulder, a runner might experience runner's knee, and a cyclist may well experience IT-band syndrome. All these occur from repetition in the same range of motion over extended periods of time. Sticking to only one sport might cause you to accidentally avoid training other muscle groups. This can lead to asymmetry, imbalance, and ultimately injury.

We are finding runners who have begun to experience knee problems and other related warning signs of overuse coming over to triathlon to experience the benefits of cross-training. Colin was primarily a runner until he discovered TRI. He didn't have fun running, but he made himself do it for the heart-health benefits. One of the main reasons he disliked going for runs was that his knees would bother him during and after a workout. He tried exercises recommended by physical therapists and doctors, but nothing seemed to work … until he discovered the bike. When he started training

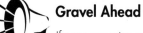

Gravel Ahead

If you experience pain or become injured, back off your training load and make some adjustments to foster recovery. Depending on the injury, you might use the RICE technique: R—rest, I—ice, C—compression, E—elevate. If your injury persists, seek medical attention.

for his first TRI, his knees started on their usual routine of pain during one of his training runs. His training mentor, Donna, told him not to worry. She said that once his bike mileage increased, his knees would get stronger and the pain would go away. She was exactly right. Now, whenever Colin hears about a runner with knee problems, his first question is "Have you tried biking?"

TRI strikes the perfect balance across the three disciplines. Moreover, if you do experience an injury, it's possible to employ cross-training principles to aid in your recovery. You usually won't have to give up your entire fitness program: you may be able to modify or substitute activities. For example, if your knee has been aching from increased running mileage, you could back off of running while increasing your swim yardage. This would give your body time to recover while maintaining current levels of cardiovascular conditioning.

Variety Is the Spice of Life

Almost everyone would prefer to be physically fit than not. Very few people wake up thinking *I'm so glad to be overweight, and I love getting out of breath when I climb the stairs*. So what keeps us from achieving this goal of health and fitness? Two major stumbling blocks: lack of motivation and/or boredom.

Sometimes the desire is there, but the thought of getting on the treadmill in the dead of winter is nauseating. This is where workouts go from a consistent 3 days a week to sporadic at best. On the other hand, there are the weekend warrior types who get together for a weekly game of basketball or volleyball. They're winded in the first 5 minutes, but they love what they're doing.

The key to fitness is consistent activity. If we could bring the two examples together, blending desire with fun, we would be in good shape. We are pretty sure there might be a sport out there that does this. What is it again? Oh yeah, *triathlon!* It offers variety, challenge, and fun. TRI goes beyond the sports of swimming, biking, and running. Many who train for triathlons also incorporate strength training, yoga, and Pilates workouts. This comprehensive approach adds flavor and spice to each day.

Taking it a step further, you'll seek to find novel methods of carrying out each activity. For example, if you live by the ocean, you can substitute a half-hour of body surfing for your lap workout. Swimming out through the waves and riding them back to the beach mimics interval training: high intensity going out and recovery on the way back in. And it's a blast!

Inner Peace: Finding Zen

We live in a busy world with many distractions. Some days feel full of chaos, packed with stress, worry, and grief. We're not saying TRI is a universal panacea for all the world's troubles. However, TRI comes with countless advantages that can improve your quality of life. There's more than the obvious myriad health and fitness benefits TRI contributes to: there's an underlying quality that you will recognize and tap into. Some call it peace of mind: others call it Zen.

Although perhaps overused lately, *Zen* really captures the essence of this quality. Zen relies heavily on obtaining enlightenment by way of meditation, and training for TRI can be meditative at times. We are not advocating any religious belief: we are merely acknowledging the connection that can be found between TRI and Zen.

Because his umbilical cord was wrapped around his neck at birth, Rick Hoyt (left) suffered brain damage. Although he can only communicate with a special computer, he and his father, Dick (right), find true inner peace when they compete together in triathlon.

(Photo by Lois Schwartz)

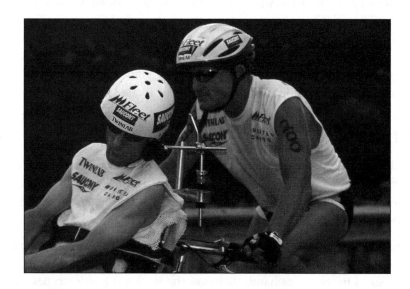

We believe that TRI teaches you to be in the present moment. When you're training or racing, you must focus on the *now* of things:

> *How's my pace?*
>
> *How's my form?*

Don't step in that pothole.

It's time to drink some water.

When your attention is in the present, you feel a stillness, a calmness, and a sense of peace. The mind is a powerful thing. TRI can help you better understand the mind-body connection and how you can use it to relax. Be in the moment!

The Social Side

TRI involves so many training possibilities, and there are just as many social interaction opportunities. You may have a different workout partner for each activity: pool swimming, open-water swimming, bike riding, trail running, yoga, and resistance training. You may meet with certain groups for certain workouts.

Spinning or other cycling classes are also great ways to be social. You might find an instructor you love or attend with some friends. These classes can be focused and intense, but there's also room for interaction and bonding.

> **Coaches' Corner**
>
> We used to meet up with an all-ages group every Wednesday morning for a long bike ride. In addition to the camaraderie of training with others, rides like this add extrinsic motivation. You're less likely to skip a session if your friends are waiting at the corner of Cross and Train.

Many triathletes get involved with local TRI clubs. This is a great way to meet people, forge relationships, learn, and have fun. Clubs may have websites with useful information about races and group events (see Appendix B). They typically get together weekly, monthly, or quarterly. Some hold mini-races and afterward offer food and drink.

> **Coaches' Corner**
>
> The Leukemia and Lymphoma Society's Team-in-Training, one of the world's largest endurance sports training organizations, helps train participants to run or walk a full or half marathon, participate in a triathlon, or complete a century (100-mile) bike ride, all while raising money for charity. Since 1988, more than 200,000 volunteers have raised more than half a billion dollars to combat leukemia and lymphoma. Team-in-Training was how Steve got his start toward endurance fitness vs. weight training. Even though he had never run more than 5 miles, he signed up for a marathon. Team-in-Training offers group workouts, coaching advise, social gatherings, and overall support. Beyond the social aspect, you are contributing to a greater good.

The TRI community has its own subculture. They look like everyone else, but typically possess many of the following characteristics: confidence, focus, adaptability, emotional stability, and mental toughness. Triathletes have the "anything is possible" attitude. Steve will never forget when he was just getting into this sport. He went down to an ocean cove with his workout partner for a swim at 5 o'clock on a Friday. It was his first time there, and he couldn't believe his eyes. Scores of people on the lawn above the cove were getting suited up for a swim. They had their towels, wetsuits, and goggles. Steve kept telling himself it was a Friday after work. He thought to himself, *Don't these people know about happy hour?*

This doesn't mean triathletes don't party or know how to have fun. It just means that many of them have a different method of prioritization.

A True Mind-Body-Spirit Connection

Health is made up of five main components:

- Physical
- Emotional
- Mental
- Spiritual
- Social

When we are firing on all cylinders, we have the greatest level of life quality, happiness, and self-actualization. TRI has the potential to improve each of the five facets of health. We've already discussed some of the physical, mental, and social aspects, but how does TRI affect emotional and spiritual health?

Emotion can come into play during training and competition when we are faced with struggle, accomplishment, pain, completion, fear, and doubt. Both of us have personally been brought to tears when crossing the finish line during the most difficult races and triathlons. There's an overwhelming rush of genuine emotions that can come out of nowhere. Joy, sadness, elation, relief, pride, and suffering all slam into you at once, and the tears start flowing.

The spiritual component is closely related to emotion. When we are faced with adversity, struggle, and pain, we have a propensity to look deep within for answers. We are looking for strength from our soul. It is in those times, the times we want to quit, when we push on through. It's the voice inside that cries, *Never give up!* When we learn we can tap into this inner power, we grow, evolve, and discover a truer version of ourselves. This may happen during training for or racing in any distance of TRI in which you really have to push yourself.

> **Coaches' Corner**
>
> The bottom line is that this amazing sport has the ability to cultivate introspection and self-belief. Awaken the champion inside you!

It's Okay *Not* to Race

Those who are just getting their feet wet in the sport (pun intended) may not want to enter a competition right away. That's okay. There's no rule that says training for triathlon must include signing up for a race. Maybe you just want to take your time with the sport and simply train, meet some workout partners, and join a club. You'll reap most of the same benefits as those who do an official triathlon.

Without having a specific race to train for, your challenge is setting your own goals and milestones. As a rule of thumb, shoot for one to three goals. Having just one goal can keep things focused and moving forward, but having more than three can cause confusion. Ask yourself what you want to accomplish. Take as much time as you need, and remember that you can make adjustments down the road if need be. Here are some random examples:

- Swim for *X* laps in the pool without stopping

- Bike for *X* minutes followed by an *X*-minute run

- Swim for *X* minutes straight in open water

- Work up to *X* minutes of swimming, biking, and running in succession

Regardless of what your goal is, just having one is a great start. Once you have your goal(s) in mind, assign a completion date (for example, I want to complete a *Master's swim workout* by May 15). This is a measurable objective. Now you have something concrete to strive for and accomplish.

def•i•ni•tion

A **Master's swim workout** is one that is organized and coached, with specific goals. One day may focus on intervals while the next emphasizes endurance. These workouts are also very beneficial because they typically include advice on technique.

Once you figure out your goals, write them down and display them. Whether on your fridge, by your alarm clock, or posted on your desk at the office, this visual aid will help keep you motivated and remind you of what you've mentally declared. It's especially good on days when you're having trouble keeping to a workout. Sometimes we need such a tool to give us a little nudge.

It doesn't matter if you have 12 races on your schedule or 0. In life, we all have different levels of responsibilities, free time, and personal goals. The sport of TRI can be matched to your individual needs. The most important things are to train smart, be safe, have fun, and know you can accomplish *anything* you desire.

The Least You Need to Know

- Triathlon (TRI) is relatively a young sport, starting in 1974.

- To get the most out of TRI, embrace the challenge and enjoy the journey.

- Cross-training helps you maintain your interest and reduces the chance of injury.

- Triathlon encompasses physical, mental, social, emotional, and spiritual aspects.

- Base your goals on your individual needs: races are not the end-all-be-all.

Choose Your Race Wisely

In This Chapter

◆ Checking out the five standard triathlon distances

◆ Selecting a race for you

◆ Forming a race strategy and other considerations

◆ Race locales where you can choose to race

Your big choices when it comes to race selection are distance and location. Shorter races might be as little as 6 total miles, whereas Ironman races are 140.6 total miles. Beginners typically start off with the lower-mileage races to get a feel for the sport and the time commitment necessary to succeed. People who want to do a race ASAP might want to choose a lower-mileage race as well, as you need fewer weeks to prepare.

Location is a big decision for two factors: how far will you need to travel, and what sort of weather will you find as you go? You must choose, but choose wisely.

What Are My Options?

Triathlons are made up of any three sports combined into one event. The majority of TRIs are made up of swimming, biking, and running. Swimming is generally the shortest distance, and biking is the longest, but TRIs can be made up of any distance.

For our purposes, we focus on five main distances:

- *Super-sprint:* approximately 7 miles

- *Sprint:* approximately 10 miles

- *Olympic distance:* 31.1 miles

- *Half-Ironman:* 70.3 miles

- *Ironman:* 140.6 miles

If this is your first TRI, you might want to err on the side of caution and go for a race that might be a little shorter instead of going for one that might be too long. There's nothing worse than putting unnecessary pressure on yourself to compete in a race for which you don't have ample preparation time. To that end, we wrote the following sections from the perspective of the level of experience necessary to conquer your first race. This doesn't mean you won't be able to take on one of the longer races in your first season, but you might want to complete a shorter race to prepare for a longer one.

Another reason to start off with a shorter race is to build your confidence. If your end goal is a longer race, completing a shorter-distance TRI helps you gain a sense of accomplishment and knowledge that you *can* finish.

Athletes of all ages, ability, and personal challenges conquer triathlons. This athlete is paralyzed from the waist down but finds success in triathlon.

(Photo by Lois Schwartz)

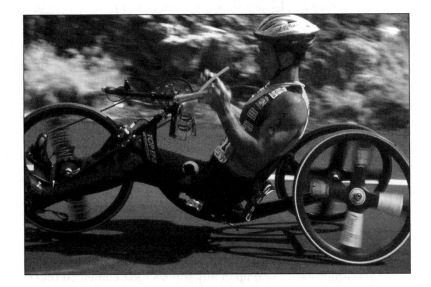

Super-Sprint

This is probably the shortest standard triathlon distance you'll find. Sample distances include the following:

- *Swim:* 300 meters to 500 meters (0.19 miles to 0.31 miles)

- *Bike:* 10 kilometers to 16 kilometers (6 miles to 10 miles)

- *Run:* 1 kilometer to 3 kilometers (0.62 miles to 1.86 miles)

These races are great for triathletes who don't have time to train too much (or don't want to), don't feel fully confident in one or more of the three sports, or are just coming back from an injury.

As you can imagine, with the distances in this race being so short, you better get warmed up before the gun goes off. After that starting pistol fires, you will be constantly moving until you cross the finish line.

Training Tips

In a super-sprint triathlon, you won't need to take in any calories. You will get by just fine with a few swigs of water or sport drink. Carry a bottle on your bike and use as needed.

Since the race is so short, athletes want to minimize all equipment and clothing changes between sports (their transition). For example, you'll want to wear the same jersey (with your race number already attached) throughout the entire race. If the water is warm enough, avoid a wetsuit altogether. These are just a couple things that will save you precious seconds (we cover a few more in Chapter 8).

A super-sprint triathlon can be very intense because the athletes tend to push full-out the entire time. There's very little "settling in" as there is in some of the longer distances.

This is also a perfect race for someone who wants to race as part of a vacation or a trip, as it will take up minimal time and, with proper nutrition and hydration, won't make a huge impact to the rest of your day or week.

Sprint

Sprint-distance triathlons are a bit longer than super-sprints, but there is no clear line drawn to distinctly divide the two. Possible distances for sprint distance would be the following:

- *Swim:* 375 meters to 750 meters (0.23 miles to 0.47 miles)

- *Bike:* 10 kilometers to 22 kilometers (6.2 miles to 13.2 miles)

- *Run:* 3 kilometers to 5 kilometers (1.9 miles to 3.1 miles)

Coaches' Corner

Sprint races are more common than super-sprint, and most local races offer this distance. This was the first distance TRI Colin ever did, and for him, it was not too long … not too short … it was just right.

This is also a great first race distance. The biggest obstacle that could exist with a sprint would be for a beginning swimmer and a course of 750 meters. (Lucky for you, you are reading a great guidebook that will have you completely prepared for this race!) This distance is also a nice distance for those who have had some time off and want to get back into the feel of organized triathlons or who are trying to test the recovery of an injury.

A long transition in this race could also add significantly to your total finishing time, but that shouldn't be a concern (just something you should be aware of).

The sprint can take from less than 1 hour to 2 or more hours, depending on your fitness level. It won't take up your entire day, and you should be able to recover relatively quickly with proper nutrition and hydration. The next day, your muscles might remind you that you did something out of the ordinary the day before, but you should feel minimal soreness. This is another great vacation triathlon.

Olympic

Olympic distance triathlons are exactly that: events which are the distance of the triathlon that takes place in the Olympics. The distances are standardized:

- *Swim:* 1.5 kilometers (0.9 miles)
- *Bike:* 40 kilometers (24 miles)
- *Run:* 10 kilometers (6.2 miles)

This race is more than 50 km (30 miles) long, so it's not generally for a first timer. However, it could be a first race for those of you who are willing to put in the time it takes to prepare. This is a great practice race for people who are getting ready to do a longer triathlon in the next couple weeks or a month.

The swim (as well as the other parts of the race) is too long to be fueled solely by adrenaline. This is a distance that will require proper pacing. If you go out too hard and keep up an unreasonable pace throughout the entire swim and beginning of the bike, it will negatively impact you either during the second half of the bike segment or on the run.

The number of people who need to walk during the run portion of an Olympic distance triathlon is exponentially greater than the number who need to walk during a sprint or super-sprint. Why? Because the length of each leg is not necessarily enough to intimidate, and athletes go out with a sprint mentality.

Coaches' Corner

Going out too hard happens to the best of us, and it happens repeatedly. We have seen it happen to all levels of athletes from beginners to the most elite. There is rarely an Ironman World Championship Triathlon televised that doesn't include a professional who ends up walking part or all of the end of the race in tears. The key to overcoming the "push-too-hard" curse is to be conscious that it will happen … and be prepared to reign yourself in when it does occur. When you realize that you're going faster than you had planned, just take a moment to relax and decide that you're going to deliberately slow down and settle into your pace.

This race will require you to have a plan to take in fluids and possibly fuel. (We discuss nutrition on the move in detail in Chapter 9.) You'll definitely need to stay hydrated during your Olympic-distance experience. This course could take you from less than 2 hours to upward of 4 hours, depending on your pace. You will definitely need a little more recovery time after this race than after shorter events, and your muscles will probably feel fatigued for the rest of the day. Be prepared for some soreness the next day as well.

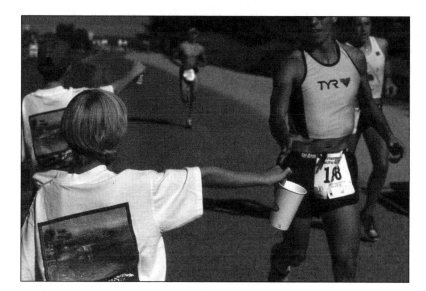

Fueling on the move can be a challenge, but with practice, you'll do it like a pro.

(Photo by Lois Schwartz)

Half-Ironman

Although the half-Ironman swim distance is only a 25 percent increase from the Olympic-distance triathlon, the bike and run portions of the half-Ironman are more than 100 percent increases in distance!

♦ *Swim:* 1.9 kilometers (1.2 miles)

♦ *Bike:* 89.6 kilometers (56 miles)

♦ *Run:* 21 kilometers (13.1 miles)

The elite athletes can finish in less than 4 hours, and the cutoff time is 8 hours and 30 minutes. Only those who are really going to be able to fully commit to their training should attempt a half-Ironman. To prepare for this race, athletes need to workout most days during the week. Your body is going to need to adapt to very long workouts.

Pacing is more than just something to keep in your head. You need to plan your pacing. Of course, you can make adjustments and listen to your body, but you should have a pretty solid idea about your pace for each leg of the triathlon before the starter's gun goes off.

Coaches' Corner

Pushing yourself too hard at the start of a race, only to lose steam later, is known in the TRI world as a "blowup" or, more commonly, "bonking." There's nothing worse than spending months training for the culmination of your season ... and then having to go half-speed for the second half of your event because you went out too hard at the beginning.

Going too hard will definitely result in your body becoming exhausted later in the race. You may want to consciously start out slower than your usual pace, and gradually increase speed as the race progresses.

You'll have time to get in a groove. You'll have time to think. You'll have time to focus and evaluate yourself during a half-Ironman. Use this time wisely. If you make a mistake early by pushing too hard or if a race official penalizes you, don't sweat it. Fix it. Relax into your pace and be sure you're following the rules. Keep a good head on your shoulders and get the job done.

Generally speaking, half-Ironman races have many spectators, volunteers, and aid stations to keep the day going smoothly for everyone involved. You will need to have a nutrition/hydration plan set in your mind before attacking this distance. Supply won't be an issue; there will be several places to grab food and drink, you'll simply need to know when, what, and how much you should be ingesting.

Ironman

This is the granddaddy of all the triathlons. Whenever the sport of TRI is discussed, this is the race that pops into most people's mind. Part of the reason it's so well known is that the world championship race is on network TV every year. The narrated stories in the TV special draw you in and leave you wondering how this race is physically possible. The distances are intimidating, to say the least:

- *Swim:* 3.8 kilometers (2.4 miles)
- *Bike:* 179.2 kilometers (112 miles)
- *Run:* 42 kilometers (26.2 miles)

You have to be a committed athlete (and probably should be committed to a psych ward!) to conquer the Ironman. Just kidding. This is usually not a first season race, but it can be done.

Ironman started as an elite challenge between about a dozen individuals, and it has grown to be the flagship of the sport. The most elite athletes can finish this race in around 8 hours, while the maximum time allotted is 17 hours. Some people don't finish in the allotted time, but still push on, finishing in 18, 19, or even 20 hours. Although they don't get the official finisher's medal, those athletes prove that they are fierce triathletes at heart.

If you want to become an Ironman triathlete, you're going to need to make serious time in your schedule for training. Even if you're a great athlete and the type of person who can just go run a marathon without training, you can't fake the Ironman. You need to fully commit yourself to this journey. You have to work out for more than an hour most days of the week, with some weekend workouts nearing the length of a standard workday! If an Ironman is your goal, you can make time for your training. *You can do this.*

Gravel Ahead _____

If you're going to become an Ironman athlete, it's very important that, before any training, you take some time to really evaluate if you're going to be able to make the time commitment. Review the training schedule (see Chapter 14) and think about your personal life and your professional life. Talk with the people who are important to you, and be sure they both understand your desire and are ready to support you in your quest.

How Long Until T-Day?

One of the biggest considerations when deciding what race you want to shoot for is how long you have until race day. If the race is coming up in a few short months, it might be tight. Will you have enough time to prepare for the distance you want to conquer? Will your work and/or life schedules allow for some adjustments in the short term? Perhaps you have many months before your goal race. With proper planning, you can make any race happen with enough time ahead of you.

It's probably easy to understand the following concept: the longer the race you're preparing for, the more time you need to train. If your goal is to compete in a sprint triathlon, you'll be able to prepare in 3 months (less if you're already in good shape and possibly more if you're really out of shape). If you want to go for the Ironman distance, you'll need about 6 months. These amounts of time can be adjusted based on your current fitness level.

Average Weeks Needed to Prepare for Triathlon

Distance	Training Time
Super-sprint	4 to 10 weeks
Sprint	6 to 14 weeks
Olympic distance	8 to 16 weeks
Half-Ironman*	10 to 20 weeks
Ironman*	16 to 30 weeks

Many triathletes wait until at least their second season of triathlon to attempt these distances.

Destination Unknown

Now that you have some idea about the race distance and the necessary time to train, you can decide where you want to compete. Most likely, you can find some races in your general area. However, they might not match your distance requirements (there are only a few Ironman distance races in the entire world). If you're looking to travel to your race, literally thousands of options around the world are available to you.

The big question is: should you stick to a location you can drive to on the day of the race, or do you want to venture out farther and accomplish your feat somewhere away from home? There are several positives and a couple negatives to either option. Let's take a deeper look.

Close to Home

Participating in a race within reasonable driving distance of your home gives you home field advantage. You're able to organize and reorganize your equipment several times the night before the race, sleep in your own bed, use your own alarm clock to wake up in the morning, and prepare whatever meals you would like in your own kitchen.

There's always a certain amount of second-guessing about equipment prep. Even after you've laid out everything you think you'll need for the next day, you'll remember something and think, *Did I remember an extra* _____*?* [fill in the blank]. If you're at home, it's easy to pop out of bed and go check. If you did forget the item, you can put it in with your gear. If you're away from home and you forgot something, you'll be S.O.L. (simply out of luck). You'll have to either complete the TRI without the missing equipment, or figure out a way to get a last-minute replacement.

There's a lot to be said about sleeping in your own bed and making food in your own kitchen. You know the sounds in your home, the softness of your mattress, and how the stove burners function. There should be very few, if any, surprises in your house. *Su casa es su casa.*

Exploring Your World

Completing a triathlon in a faraway place can be a great way to get a special perspective on a travel destination. Going to another location can make you feel more "official." Experiencing a race in a different environment/climate/etc. might help your mind focus on the big day. It somewhat removes you from other distractions and concerns that might cause worry in your home environment.

Doing a TRI away from home can also add extrinsic motivation. Because there's more cost and logistical planning associated with remote races, you'll probably feel more invested. Therefore, you'll most likely be more compelled to follow through with your training and racing.

That all said, arranging travel can add stress. If you decide that you're going to travel to some-where far from your home, there's one final decision to make: will you drive to the destination or fly? If your bike will fit in your car, no further equipment is necessary. If you're going to fly to your TRI, you need to purchase a bike box. This is a hard case that enables you to safely transport your bike in the plane's baggage hold. A bike box adds some cost (you can get them new or used), and airlines typically charge an additional cost to bring a bike on a plane. Don't forget to factor in this cost when you're making the decision to fly, and talk to someone at the airline to confirm their policy before making your reservation (see Chapter 3 for more information on bike boxes).

Training Tips _____

If you don't want to take your bike to the airport with you, you might want to look into other options. Some companies offer door-to-door bike shipping services. The prices vary depending upon the company, the distance to the race, and the degree to which you need assistance. Some services include pick up, shipping, and return while others also include bike disassembly and reassembly. Search on the web for companies near you, or check out Appendix B.

If you decide to travel away from home, most likely you'll be staying at a friend's house or at a hotel. If you're going to stay at a friend's house, be sure he or she understands how important your big day is. Be sure he or she comprehends what sort of needs you'll have the night before and the morning of your race. You'll need peace. You'll need quiet. You'll need a comfortable spot to rest and some specific breakfast food.

If you opt to stay in a hotel, book it early. Getting a spot in the race is the most important, but getting a room in a hotel is a close second. With bigger, more renowned races, you might have trouble getting into a hotel near the starting line. For the bigger races, reserve your hotel before you even sign up for the race. Be sure to confirm the hotel's cancellation policy, too. Almost all standard hotels across the country have a no-penalty cancellation policy, as long as you do it a day or two before you're supposed to arrive.

Traveling away from home might limit your food choices leading up to the race. If you're used to eating out and don't mind a restaurant for a prerace breakfast (and have tried eating out before a workout before), this might not adversely affect you. If you're used to a very specific breakfast, you should try to find a suite-style hotel so you can prepare the food yourself.

Traveling also affects how many people will be at your race to cheer you on. If you don't want anyone to come watch you show how tough you are, this won't be an issue. However, if you would appreciate some groupies to help keep you motivated, this might be a bigger decision for you to make. Even if people want to support you, they might not be able to afford the time or money to come watch your race if it's far from their home. For those who can't make it, some races have websites showing near real-time results and web-cams. Your friends and family may be able to follow you along during the race even if they're not physically there with you.

Gravel Ahead _____

Set several alarm clocks the night before your race. If you're staying in a hotel, it surely will have a clock in the room. However, have a backup in place by setting a travel alarm clock and/or watch and/or cell phone. You don't want to be the guy who shows up to the race late, after being confused the night before about the A.M./P.M. marker on an unfamiliar alarm clock.

Matching Personal Goals to a Distance

Only you know what you want to achieve. You know what you're trying to do. Would you like to train for a triathlon and not necessarily compete in one? Do you want to lose some weight and just adopt a healthier lifestyle? Do you want to complete an Olympic-distance triathlon after witnessing this in the last summer Olympics?

This is one area where we cannot offer too much advice. Only you can match your personal goal to a race distance and training schedule. People who don't really want to commit to a scheduled race and/or who are just starting out in all three sports might want to look into a sprint or Olympic-distance race/training program.

If you've already done a few sprint TRIs and are comfortable with all three sports (and of course, you have the time), you might want to consider bumping up to an Olympic distance or longer. If you already know that you like TRI, have a very flexible schedule, and really want to put in some serious hours training, think about a half-Ironman or full Ironman. Try to figure out how much time you'll have available for training per week, and compare that with the hours associated with the different training programs outlined later in the book. Only you can decide what's best for you.

> **Training Tips** _____
>
> Meditate on what you want to do in your triathlon experience. If you're carrying a few more pounds than you want, your goal might be to just get into a workout routine and the distance doesn't matter. Take some time to really decide what your goal will be, and be sure your goals match the amount of time you'll be able to commit.

Sign Up Early

If you decide that part of your goal is to do an official triathlon, you should sign up. You can do it. What's stopping you? Grab your credit card, find an Internet connection, and get it done. Make the commitment to compete in a triathlon. We've got your back. If you're brand new to the sport, you can finish the book first and then go for it.

Entry fees associated with TRI events depend on the location, distance, and other logistics, such as aid stations on the course. The range in price is vast: a short, local mini-sprint may cost you $15, while an Ironman could run you nearly 500 bucks! Some events can be paid for in advance online or with a check via good old snail mail. Many races offer a discount for those who sign up early, and same-day registration is not an option for some races. Active. com is one of the leaders in national online event registration (see Appendix B).

Once you've signed up, you're set! Well, except for all the hard work and planning still to come—but you're doing it! Mark your triathlon on the calendar in the kitchen or at the office or both, and get focused.

Another great reason to sign up early is that some races fill up quickly. Most North American Ironman races reach the maximum capacity after only a few hours of open signup! The majority of other races have registration for a significantly longer period of time, but any of them can close at any time. Don't start training and think *I'll get around to signing up eventually*. You could be in for some serious disappointment if the race you were aiming for is no longer available because of your procrastination.

Hopefully, you won't need to cancel after signing up for a race, but if you think there might be a chance, be sure you read the race cancellation policy thoroughly upfront. Some races offer a credit for cancellations that you can apply toward another event or partial refunds. Others clearly indicate, "No refunds." Be sure you understand the rules and regulations of your event.

The Least You Need to Know

- ◆ Decide if you want to attempt a race, and if so, what distance.

- ◆ Evaluate the pluses and minuses of doing a race near your home or somewhere far away.

- ◆ Factor together your goals and the time you have available before the big race to make a final decision.

- ◆ Sign up for your triathlon as early as possible.

Chapter 3

Equipment: Needs vs. Wants

In This Chapter

- ◆ Necessary TRI equipment
- ◆ Tips on selecting the gear right for you
- ◆ Upgrading your equipment arsenal

You don't need too much *stuff* to participate in triathlon. A bike, a swimsuit, and shoes are the bare necessities.

That said, it is possible to spend thousands of dollars on top-of-the-line items. Equipment is just a small part of the overall equation, though. You're still the one who needs to do the work! A fancy wetsuit won't swim for you. Expensive bikes don't pedal themselves. And you know those shoes are made for running … but they're not going to run anywhere without you.

Some people become intimidated by all the equipment choices in the TRI world. They get stressed out trying to decide between one brand and another of this or that. You won't. By the end of this chapter, you'll know what you need, and you'll know that whatever you choose will work.

The Basic Principles

The keys for selecting triathlon equipment are comfort and efficiency. If your shoes are too tight or your bike hurts your back when you ride it, you'll be less apt to continue with your training program. You have to *want* to get out there!

Efficiency is also an important factor in equipment choices. If you go running with weighty, bricklike boots on your feet, you're going to think, *running sucks!* because your feet are so heavy. Lighter, well-designed running shoes are going to make your running experience much better than shoes not intended specifically for the sport.

More efficient equipment can make your TRI experience easier and more enjoyable. Only you can decide how much each step up in efficiency is worth.

Swim

Almost everyone has a swimsuit somewhere in his or her wardrobe. It may not be sleek and it may not be stylish but that doesn't matter. You really don't need much before you jump in and get your feet wet.

The Bare Necessities

Any swimsuit that fits you and any pair of goggles that don't leak will enable you to participate in warmer water triathlons.

Swimsuit   The swimsuit can be loose or tight, big or small, one piece or two. That said, most people who swim for fitness and training will choose to wear a one-piece, form-fitting suit. This enables you to cut through the water more efficiently.

A tighter suit also allows your swim instructor (if you have a coach or go to a Master's class) to see your form more easily as he or she is critiquing your overall technique. Helpful tips and small corrections in your form will definitely cause your time to improve both in the swim (you'll be moving faster) and in the rest of your triathlon (you'll have wasted less energy in the water).

Training Tips

Keep in mind that everyone's face is shaped differently. What might be the perfect pair of goggles for one person might not even form a seal over another person's eyes. If you have the opportunity to try out a friend's goggles before you buy your own, go for it.

Goggles   Goggles are the other necessity for swimming. A nice pair of goggles aren't very expensive and are a great investment that will make your experiences in the pool much better. Beyond keeping water out of your eyes, you want the goggles to be comfortable and you don't want them to pinch in any spots.

Many anti-fog variety goggles are available, but if you don't get that type, just rub a little spit on the lenses before you put them on in the water and you'll be golden. We each went through three pairs before we found the right fit. Now that we know what works, we keep a backup pair in our swim bag in case one breaks or our current pair goes missing.

Wetsuit   If you'll be training or competing in cooler water, you'll most likely need a wetsuit. (This last "bare necessity," might be in your "add-on" category, depending on your goal.) If the temperature doesn't force you to wear a wetsuit, you might still want to consider it, as it will add buoyancy and efficiency. You'll notice the increased buoyancy; you might not notice the efficiency, but trust us … it is there.

Triathletes use two main types of wetsuits:

- *Full* covers your core and extends down your arms to your wrists and down your legs to your ankles.

- *Sleeveless* is simply an armless full.

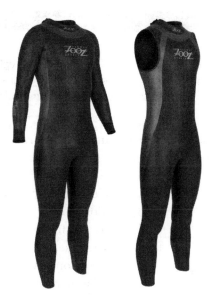

The best type of wetsuit for you depends on how much warmth you want and how comfortable you feel in either of the options.

(Courtesy of Zoot Sports)

When you try on a wetsuit, it should feel tight. You don't want it to cut off circulation, but you don't want to have "room to grow," either. Most people feel slightly uncomfortable when they first put one on … and possibly again after a big holiday dinner. You'll get used to it after a few swims. We know some triathletes who opt for the sleeveless version because it feels less constricting to them. It's all about your personal preference.

Lubrication   If you do purchase a wetsuit, lubrication becomes a "bare necessity" as well. The motions of swimming while in a wetsuit will cause your body to rub against the suit and could cause serious chaffing. Even the simple movement of turning your head to breathe while swimming in a wetsuit can cause irritation on the back of your neck after only a few minutes. Use some lubrication to cover these areas. We get into more lube details in the "Other Equipment" section of this chapter, but *do not* forget to use it with a wetsuit. We've seen triathletes use deodorant or even cooking spray to reduce the rub. Who said triathletes weren't creative?

Gravel Ahead

Be sure to use some kind of lubricant if you wear a wetsuit, but be careful what kind you choose. Petroleum-based products can degrade wetsuit material and are not recommended.

Add-Ons

Both men and women can wear trisuits, one-piece singlets that cover their entire body. These can be worn in warm water as a swimsuit and then stay on during both the bike and the run.

Trisuits wick water away from your skin and bring it to the surface of the suit to get you dry as quickly as possible. (You'll find that most TRI gear "wicks" water away.)

Coaches' Corner
Although a trisuit is the epitome of efficiency, it might not be as comfortable as bike shorts while riding because the butt cushion (chamois) is typically a little thinner. If you're thinking about using a trisuit in a race, be sure you try it ahead of time. Let your butt decide. One more thing: bathroom breaks can become a little more … interesting.

Certain arms-only or legs-only drills during swim training necessitate you to have a way to keep half of your body immobile but afloat as you swim across the pool. Pull buoys and kickboards do just that. You can squeeze a pull buoy between your thighs to keep your legs near the surface as you focus on specific upper body techniques. Kickboards keep your upper body afloat during leg drills. Although the pool where you decide to swim may already have these pieces of equipment for general use, some people prefer to bring their own. If you go this route, write your name on the equipment with a permanent marker.

Gravel Ahead

Several variations of these buoys and kickboards are available. Some look like futuristic, aerodynamic spaceships, and others just look like a piece of foam. The boring-looking pull buoy or kickboard does the exact same job, usually for much less cost. Don't be fooled by fancy looks and packaging when it comes to swimming aids.

Hand paddles and fins might also be helpful in your training, but definitely aren't necessary. Swimming with paddles on your hands and/or with fins on your feet enables you to increase the surface area where you're pushing against the water and, therefore, increase the power necessary to move forward. They increase your speed and make you feel the water sliding by you much faster. Neither of these is allowed in races, as it would give an unfair advantage, but both can be used to augment your training program.

Supplementing Your Gear

If money is no object, you should definitely investigate a couple options that give you a lap lane in your backyard or indoors: a "never-ending" pool and a current maker. Both options essentially allow you to swim in place like a water treadmill. Check online for more information if this is something you're interested in (and can afford).

Bike

For the bike portion of a triathlon, you'll need a bike—a mountain bike, road bike, or even a dirt bike for shorter races. However, cycling can become the most equipment-heavy aspect of TRI in a hurry. If you want to be more efficient and comfortable, you can always pick up a few additional items. Some will make you more aerodynamic; others enable you to use your leg muscles more fully. Your end goals will help determine how far you should go with the extras.

The Bare Necessities

The obvious, most important thing that you need for this leg of triathlon is a bicycle.

Bike   If you're already physically fit and you're looking to do an extremely short TRI like a super-sprint, a one-speed bike might suffice. However, we definitely recommend one with several speeds, and if you conquer just one hill with it, you'll understand why. The big front chain ring–small rear chain ring combo enables you to pedal with serious power. Flying down a hill is the perfect opportunity to use this. When you're climbing back up the hill, the small front chain ring–big rear chain ring combo will enable you to get extreme efficiency out of each pedal rotation.

Helmet—*Not* an Optional Piece of Equipment   A helmet is not a discussion point. Get one. Get it before you go out for any ride. We don't care if you think helmets are only for kids with overprotective parents. You are no longer going to be riding around the block on the sidewalk; you're becoming a triathlete. You'll be out on the street with traffic around you, and you'll be going at speeds you may not have reached before on a bike. A helmet could save your life in an accident.

Almost all bike helmets are not multi-impact helmets; they need to be replaced after one serious impact. Most manufacturers encourage bikers to replace a helmet that's been dropped on the ground or been in a small crash, because deficiencies in the helmet may exist without being visible. Whatever helmet you choose to use, be sure it's certified by the U.S. Consumer Product Safety Commission (CPSC). Check the label or box for this certification.

Pedals   Beyond the frame, two wheels, handlebars, seat (also called a saddle), and helmet, you should really consider starting off with at least a minor pedal upgrade. Having flat, standard pedals without any way to attach your foot only enables you to generate power on the down stroke. To truly be efficient, you ideally want to be able to move your feet in a circle, instead of just pushing down every pedal revolution. Pedal straps or toe clips are relatively cheap and add a great deal of efficiency because you can push down, push forward, and pull up with your legs as the pedals rotate around the crank. We go into the physics of it all a bit more in Chapter 6.

Coaches' Corner

Some evidence has shown that having a bottle cage in the back is more aerodynamic. However, any advantage is miniscule and shouldn't be the deciding factor for most age groupers.

Water Bottle Holders   Depending on how far you're going in training, you'll probably want to have some sort of water bottle cage (holder) on your bike. Most people need to drink a single, 24-ounce (710-mL) bottle of liquid during an hour of biking.

You can mount cages in a couple different ways: inside your frame or behind your saddle. Would you rather reach down or behind to get the bottle? If you're going to be out for long rides where you'll need several bottles, you might need both.

In Case of a Flat ...   A spare tube and an inflation device need to be on your "must-have" list. A tube only costs a few dollars, and a mini-pump that attaches to your bike shouldn't cost much more. There's absolutely nothing worse than being halfway done with a ride, about to turn around, and then have a tire go flat with no spare tube to fix it. A fellow rider might be able to save the day, or a cell phone could allow you to phone a friend, but you'd be better off just being prepared from the start. Also, you'll probably want to have a full-size pump at home to pump up your tires before and after your rides. Be sure to bring an Allen wrench if your wheels don't have a quick release lever.

Sunglasses   You shouldn't ride without sunglasses. Beyond blocking the sun's harmful UV (ultraviolet) rays, they also keep your eyes safe in other ways. As you ride, you can get up to higher speeds than you might expect. Even an average rider can easily get up to 30 miles per hour (48 kilometers per hour) going down a long hill. Your eyes must be protected when you're going at that speed. Besides just wind, the passing car tires could send small pebbles flying, or a kamikaze horsefly might decide it's his time to go. Don't let them take your eye! Be sure the glasses you select fully cover your eyes and block UV rays.

Add-Ons

Clipless pedals and bike shoes improve your efficiency greatly, because your bike shoe is secured to a cleat and snapped into the pedal (like a ski boot in its binding). This enables you to truly move your foot in a circular motion and use every possible directional muscle in your leg to power your ride. Plus, you won't have to worry about your foot slipping out of a strap anymore.

When you go this route, you incur two expenses: the bike shoe, and the cleat/pedal combination. A couple different versions are available; check with your local bike shop. If you opt for clipless pedals, be sure to practice snapping into and out of the pedals several times before heading out in traffic.

One of the best upgrades you can make to the cycling portion of the TRI is a bike computer. The most basic computers keep track of speed, distance, and time. For a few dollars more, you can get one that also shows your pedals' rotations per minute (RPM). If you decide to get a computer, we recommend you be sure it has this feature.

A seat pack and/or a Bento Box are great for carrying small pieces of equipment or food while out on a ride. A seat pack attaches below and behind the seat and usually has room for a spare tube, a bike tool, and some spare cash. It is also a great spot to stash your cell phone if you don't want to carry it in a pocket. Typically, a Bento Box sits on your top bike tube, just behind the handlebars. It is secured by some Velcro straps and has less space than the seat pack. Bento Boxes are a great place to carry some energy gels or bars. Neither of these items should cost very much, and both offer loads of convenience.

Aerodynamic handlebars, or aero bars, are a great addition for any cyclist who will be riding long stretches on relatively flat terrain, as they can add both a level of comfort and efficiency. (Aero bars are not used when riding in a close pack or when going up long inclines.)

Aero bars are a combination of handlebars and elbow supports that enable you to get your head and shoulders lower and more forward than you can with regular handlebars. Ideally, your elbows will be close to right angles, and most of the weight from your head and shoulders will transfer straight through your upper arms into the elbow supports. The lower your upper body, the more aerodynamic you become. Although you may not notice a change on a short ride on a windless day, the benefits will be very evident on a long ride or anytime the wind is in your face.

Aero bars are either "extensions" (a piece added to your standard handlebars that allows you to get aero) or "integrated" (the aero bars replace your standard bars, and leave you without a "drop" section on the bars). No matter which way you go, be sure you're properly fitted before making any purchase.

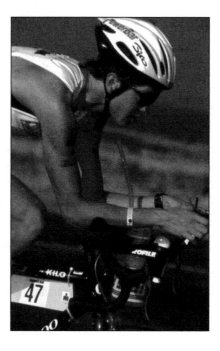

Utilizing aero bars makes you more streamlined and helps minimize the effects of headwinds.

(Photo by Lois Schwartz)

Hopefully, you'll be able to do most of your biking outside, but an indoor bike trainer can be very helpful when the great outdoors is too cold, hot, wet, or dark. It can also be used to do specific workouts in a controlled environment. These little devices elevate the back wheel of your bike and apply resistance to the tire. You can then ride and ride and get a great workout … without going anywhere. The resistance can be applied by a fan, magnet, or fluid. Fan indoor trainers are at the lower end of the price range but can get very loud. Magnet trainers are much quieter and not much more expensive than fan versions. The most expensive type of trainer, with fluid resistance, produces less heat buildup on your tires (and, therefore, less wear).

A smaller bike seat and bike shorts can help your legs be more efficient. These shorts are made of a leg-hugging material that not only reduces wind resistance, but also wicks away sweat. The most important thing, however, is that bike shorts have a pad (called a chamois) that cushions your butt from some of the pain you might experience from a smaller, harder seat than you're used to. The shorts might feel a bit uncomfortable at first, but trust us, everyone is wearing them.

Training Tips

Although it might not be intuitive, don't wear underwear underneath the bike shorts.

When most people first get bike shorts, they elect to get a matching jersey. A jersey assists in *wicking* and aerodynamics like the shorts and has the added bonus of one to three pockets. These pockets come in very handy when you need to carry snacks, cell phones, or anything else out on a ride. And although it may seem awkward to have pockets on your back at first, you'll get used to it in no time.

def•i•ni•tion

Clothing that becomes wet from sweat and/or water can be uncomfortable and cause chaffing. In fitness-clothing-speak, **wicking** is the process by which sweat is drawn away from the skin and to the outside of clothing to keep the skin dry. Clothing that wicks is also less likely to cause chafing.

CO_2 cartridges and a regulator valve are two things that can make changing a flat a little less painful. The CO_2 cartridge is a single use cylinder, only a few inches long, that attaches to the small regulator valve. When inflating, you put the other end of the valve device on your tire valve, and use the compressed gas to rapidly inflate your tire.

The cartridge will get cold, and the air in the tire will be warm. As the gas in the tire cools, it will decrease in pressure slightly, so be sure to check the pressure when you get home.

Bike gloves are another option. They have some padding around the palms to cushion your hands and cutoff fingers so you can still be dexterous. Some triathletes feel gloves add a level of comfort, but others don't use them at all. It's all a matter of personal preference.

Supplementing Your Gear

As with the swim section, there is always more gear you can get to add to your TRI arsenal:

◆ Upgraded bike computers that offer more than the standards, such as a GPS (global positioning system) and/or altimeter.

◆ Fancy water bottles or hydration systems that enable you to drink while in the aero position.

◆ Race wheels that are lighter and more aerodynamic; thick-rimmed (or deep-dish), three- or four-spoke, and disc are the main options.

◆ Teardrop shaped helmets for more aerodynamics.

> **Training Tips**
>
> Although altimeters and GPS locators can be interesting to have on a bike computer, don't fall victim to information overload. Only worry about the important numbers like your RPMs.

Run

Running takes the least amount of equipment. You. Shoes. Road. That's the minimum.

The Bare Necessities

When you were a kid, you probably ran with whatever shoes you had on that day, without a single thought about cushioning, stability, and durability. Without the right gear, your body probably didn't respond as well as it could have. We're going to help you learn what you need and how to get it so your upcoming runs are comfortable and fun.

To run, you need running shoes. Not gym shoes. Not basketball shoes. Definitely not bowling shoes. *Running shoes.* And the shoes don't have to break the bank. Your local department store might have specials on great running shoes from time to time, but especially if you are brand new to running, you should seriously consider going to a specialty running store for your first pair of shoes. That way, one of the experts who works there can point you to a shoe that works with your foot shape, length, and running style.

At the most basic level, be sure any shoe you choose is snug but not tight. You should have about a thumb's width of "room to grow" from your toe to the end of the shoe. You want to be able to wiggle your toes a bit and definitely don't want the end of your big toe rubbing against the tip of the shoe. The back of your foot should feel secure in the shoe as well. When you walk around, you don't

> **Training Tips**
>
> Your feet can swell up from your day's activities, so it's a good idea to shop for your shoes at the end of the day, when your feet are at their largest.

want your heel lifting away from the shoe. A shoe like this won't give you adequate support and will probably cause serious blisters on the back of your ankle.

Two other aspects to consider when making a shoe purchase are the shape of your foot (what type of arch do you have, how wide is your foot, etc.) and the biomechanics of your foot strike and push off. Many people have not considered either of these things when making a shoe purchase; and many choose instead based on style. A specialty running store employee might be able to evaluate both your foot type and running style and recommend a shoe that will compensate for any small issues and work with your foot shape and mechanics.

When evaluating you for a shoe, an expert will tell you that you are either a *pronator*, a *supinator*, or a *neutral* roller. Runners with severe overpronation or oversupination probably won't be able to compensate with just a shoe. These athletes might experience ankle or knee pain. If this happens to you, it might be time to visit the foot doctor for corrective orthotics. All serious triathletes/runners either have orthotics or have been evaluated and told they do not need them.

def•i•ni•tion

> **Pronation** occurs if your foot strikes the ground, rolls inward and forward, and then pushes off the ball of your foot/big toe. **Supination** occurs if your foot strikes the ground, rolls outward toward the outside of the foot, and then off the front-middle area of your foot/toes. A **neutral** roll occurs when you strike and then roll through the middle of your foot and off the middle/front section of your foot.

Add-Ons

A running hat can really make your running more comfortable. Try to get a hat specific for running, instead of an old baseball or trucker hat you might find in the closet. Because of their sweatbandlike lining and their ability to wick sweat, running hats keep sweat out of your eyes and keep your head cool. Additionally, most running hats are light colored on top to reflect sunlight and dark colored on the underside of the brim to absorb it. The reflection helps keep you cool, and the absorption reduces brightness in your eyes (like a baseball or football player with black stripes under his or her eyes).

Running shorts are a great addition to any runner's wardrobe. They are extremely light, come with a built-in liner (no undies required!), and many have a small inner pocket large enough to hold a key, an energy gel pack, or some emergency cash. Running shorts are so comfortable that once you start wearing them, you'll never go back to any other shorts for running again. And as with most fitness apparel, most types of shorts wick sweat away from your body.

Sick of tying your shoes? Get a lace lock. You just thread both your laces through this small plastic device, and it pinches your laces together so they're locked in place. When you need to take off the shoe, just squeeze the lock and loosen the laces. Lace locks are extremely cheap and can be found at any specialty running store and most general sports stores. One caveat: if you're an overpronator, these might not be for you. The lace locks don't offer the same degree of support as regularly tied shoestrings.

Supplementing Your Gear

There's very little equipment you truly need for running, but there is one big purchase you could make to supplement your training: a treadmill. There are many benefits to running outside, but treadmills also have their place in a workout regiment. If you have the space and the means to set one up—as well as the confidence that you'll continue to use it for a long time—a good treadmill could be a great addition.

Other Equipment

Beyond the basics necessary for swim/bike/run, a few other things will be useful in more than one of the three sports. This list is not all-inclusive, but you'll find it is definitely a good starting point.

The Bare Necessities

Some of the following equipment might seem obvious, and you might have already listed them on your shopping list, but others you might read and think, *Yeah! I wouldn't have thought of that. Thanks, TRI Guys!*

Socks   You're going to need some socks for both biking and running. It's worth paying a little more to get the thin, breathable, wicking type of sock. Stay away from cotton if possible, as that material may lead to blisters very quickly. Athletic socks are commonly made up of contents such as olefin, nylon, Spandex, and wool and can be found in any TRI, running, or cycling store.

Sunscreen   Sunscreen is a must. Unless you're going to be doing all your training and competing indoors, you should get a good bottle of sunscreen. Be sure you get one that's water and/or sweat resistant. Oftentimes, these bottles are marked "Sport." Don't try to save a buck on a bottle and get the cheap stuff, as that lotion might not absorb into your skin as easily as the nongeneric variety. Be sure to reapply as necessary. You might have to get a couple bottles per season to keep yourself protected.

Lubrication   You shouldn't try to live without lubrication, as chafing is a harsh reality for triathletes. The cost is minimal, and the pain it can save you is priceless. Spots where lube can protect you include but are not limited to the following:

- Underarms (while running or in a wetsuit)
- Back and side of the neck (while in a wetsuit)
- Thighs (while running or on the bike)

- Crotch (while running or on the bike)

- Butt (where your cheeks touch the seat)

- Nipples (while running)

A few companies package sports lubrications like deodorant sticks, which are very convenient to use. You can find these at almost any running, biking, or general sports store.

Bike Luggage   If you're going to be traveling on a plane to a race (or any plane trip where you want to bring your bike), a bike box is a necessity. The idea of a bike box is simple: to protect your bike as it's being tossed around by baggage handlers and conveyer belts. Many styles of bike boxes are available, but the concept is always the same: remove the wheels, handlebars, and seat and systematically place them into a protective case for transport. Check out the different styles online or at your local bike shop.

Gravel Ahead

If you purchase a new bike rack, before the day you plan to use it, be sure it works with your type of automobile. Hatchback cars sometimes don't get along with standard bike racks. Don't wait until the last minute to test it!

If you're traveling by car to a training location or a race, a vehicle-mounted bike racking system might be in order. Many bikes have quick-release wheels and can fit into many trunks, but if you don't want to mess with the wheel, get a bike rack. They're relatively cheap and enable you to pop your bike on and off quickly and easily. Remember to secure your bike both with bungee cords and some sort of locking device.

Cold-Weather Gear   Cold-weather gear will be necessary if you're planning to bike or run outside in the cold. Arm warmers, leg warmers, bike pants, and running vests all help keep you warm on those cold days. Arm warmers (tight material that goes from your wrist to your upper arm) are especially convenient when you're starting your ride in an early morning chill but the forecast says it'll warm up later. As soon as the temperature heats up, you can simply slide the warmers down your arms and stick them in a back pocket, all without slowing down.

No matter what cold-weather gear you get, be sure the material will wick away sweat. And if it's really cold out, remember to layer.

Watch   If you don't already have a digital watch with a stopwatch, you should try to get one. Most of your workouts are done on a timed basis, so a stopwatch is invaluable. Some models offer the ability to keep track of intermediate split times, which is nice to have but probably not necessary. Try to get a model that has a resin/rubber strap, as apposed to cloth/Velcro, as there will be less of a chance for bacteria to build up as you sweat during your workouts.

Add-Ons

A heart-rate monitor is a great addition to any triathlete's arsenal. Monitoring your pace/energy output via the heart rate is a great, time-tested method to successful training. You'll first have to understand your heart rate zones, but self-testing for those is not too difficult. (See "Managing Heart-Rate Zones" in Chapter 4 for more info on determining and staying in your target zones.) The monitor itself consists of a sensor and strap that wraps around your chest. It then sends a signal to a watch receiver you wear on your wrist. With this simple monitor, you can tell the time, date, and how fast your heart is working to keep you moving.

A TRI bag helps you get organized on your way to a race (or anytime you need to carry all your TRI equipment with you). This backpack has specific compartments for shoes, helmet, wetsuit, etc. Mesh compartments on the outside of the bag can hold any wet gear apart from your other equipment. It's got sections for everything and can really help you organize your gear before leaving the house. A TRI bag enables you to easily tote all your gear on your back, if you choose to ride your bike to a triathlon (a regular backpack could work, too).

Hydration Belt   You might also decide to invest in a strap-on hydration system, either a bladder or belt style. The bladder option consists of some sort of bag you can strap around your waist or wear on your back. The bag contains a bladder for hydration fluid, with a hose that can reach to your mouth. It's nice to always have fluids available, but the spot where the bag rests on your body will heat up and might chafe as it rubs against you. Be sure to lube up and add a lot of ice to the bladder on a hot day!

Fuel Belt   Nutrition belts, or fuel belts, are another piece of equipment you might want to consider for your runs. Most fuel belts hold multiple small plastic bottles. The bottles, which can be filled with energy gel or concentrated energy drink, are placed in holsters on the belt, and sit on the hips during the run. A fuel belt really becomes beneficial when run workouts last longer than an hour and a half or a couple hours. If you're doing an Olympic-distance race or shorter, you'll be just fine without it.

Race Belt   A race belt can be helpful in any race where you'll be wearing a race number (race bib). This number can be safety-pinned to your jersey very easily. However, a race belt allows you to attach the bib to an elastic belt, which then clips around your waist. Some triathletes prefer the race belt because they can move the bib around their upper body by adjusting the belt.

There's a plethora of gear available for TRI. We recommend starting simple with a focus on comfort and safety. You can always make additions as you discover your own idiosyncrasies. Just remember, your body and mind, not your equipment, make you a successful triathlete.

The Least You Need to Know

◆ You *need* a swimsuit, goggles, a bike, helmet, sunglasses, sunscreen, and running shoes to train for a triathlon.

◆ A wetsuit, bike computer, pedal straps (or clip-in pedals), and a hydration system will definitely help the cause.

◆ Don't blow a ton of cash on big-ticket items (treadmill, "never-ending" pool, etc.) until you're sure you'll stick with TRI.

Chapter 4

Start Your Engines

In This Chapter

- Understanding the science behind training
- Taking it easy and staying injury free
- Learning how to manage and apply training principles
- Knowing yourself

It's important to understand the basics before starting a training program. What you learn up front can save you the risk of frustration, burnout, overtraining, and injury. Not to mention that an efficient approach can save you time—a very precious commodity.

Start off slow and don't ever worry about how fast your workout partner is exercising—this is especially true if you're just starting to work out after an extended period of time off. Don't worry about how well or fast anyone else is doing; worry about you, and you'll be fine. Take your time to learn the basics about the glorious world of triathlon.

Always Consult a Doctor ...

Health screening is a critical first step to consider before entering into any training program. It's always better to err on the side of caution. With the proper modifications, almost everyone can and should engage in physical activity.

We recommend that everyone see a doctor before starting on a new and challenging workout regime. If you already know you have an increased risk for injury for one reason or another, be sure your physician addresses that concern specifically. Although many people choose to blow it off, you'll definitely be safer if you obtain a physician's release before engaging in your training program.

Other variables that can impact exercise risk include the following: health history, medications used, and lifestyle factors. You should look at the whole picture before beginning a program. Your physician can guide you.

Understanding Physiology

Now, do your best to stick with us in the upcoming pages if you're interested in the semi-scientific side of things. We'll try to strike the perfect balance between explaining the scientific processes going on in our bodies and not going too far overboard. Hang in there!

def•i•ni•tion

ATP (adenosine triphosphate) is a molecule required for your body's energy production. It can be produced both aerobically and anaerobically. **Mitochondria** are subcellular structures the body's cells need to change units of food into energy sources.

Let's look at the most basic element of life—energy. Our body's energy source is a substance called *ATP (adenosine triphosphate)*. Everything from getting in the car, to washing dishes, to a single wink of the eye requires it. Our muscle cells store a limited amount of ATP, so to maintain movement, we must replenish ATP from three possible sources:

◆ Aerobic system

◆ Anaerobic glycolysis

◆ Creatine phosphate system

The primary source of fuel for the aerobic system is fat (fatty acids) and carbohydrates (glucose). The aerobic system is the dominant source of energy when adequate oxygen meets production needs. (Aerobic means "with oxygen.") Most cells in the body contain structures called *mitochondria*, the sites where ATP is produced. The more of them we have in a cell, the better our energy production capability becomes.

When the body doesn't have sufficient oxygen, it kicks into anaerobic ("without oxygen") function, and ATP production occurs inside the cell, but outside the mitochondria, utilizing the anaerobic glycolosis and/or creatine phosphate systems—both of which are far less efficient than the aerobic system. However, when we exceed certain intensity limits, the body calls on our anaerobic systems for ATP. The level at which this occurs is called the *anaerobic threshold* or *lactate threshold*. This system cannot be maintained for long periods of time.

The primary source of anaerobic ATP production is glucose. The other source is creatine phosphate. Creatine phosphate is a molecule that can be easily and quickly broken down to produce ATP. Unfortunately, both anaerobic systems lack staying power: fatigue occurs in only seconds to minutes.

Aerobic capacity is an important component to the measure of physical fitness. It's the amount of oxygen the body can consume at max levels of endurance exercise. It's also known as *VO₂max*. This translates into volume in milliliters of oxygen used per kilogram of body weight per minute (ml/kg/min). VO_2max depends on two factors: cardiac output (Q) and the ability to extract oxygen from the blood and use it by the mitochondria:

$$Q = \text{heart rate} \times \text{stroke volume}$$

Stroke volume is the amount of blood pumped from each ventricle each time the heat beats. It is largely determined by genetics such as size of the heart, blood/hemoglobin content, mitochondria concentrations, and muscle fiber makeup. To a certain degree, training has been shown to enhance aerobic capacity.

Lactate threshold (LT) refers to the level of exercise intensity whereby lactate begins to rapidly accumulate in the blood faster than it can be metabolized. It is at this point that you can feel that burning sensation—like battery acid flowing through your legs! When this occurs, you must slow down and give your body a chance to process the lactate. Over time and with proper training, you can reduce the lactate level relative to a given pace or power. In other words, with steady exercise, running at the same speed you did last month will produce less of the fatigue causing lactate. Moreover, your tolerance for dealing with lactate can also improve.

When looking at overall fitness measurements, it's important to take into account both VO_2max and lactate threshold. If your VO_2max is high but you fatigue quickly, then performance drops. The goal is to aim for high levels of both factors to create optimum performance. Long-term training improves both systems.

Common Injuries and Prevention

Proper technique, comfortable and suitable equipment, and sufficient recovery time will help you avoid injuries. Other safeguards include gradually increasing volume, flexibility, and balanced muscular strength.

The greatest challenge we face while training is knowing the difference between normal training discomfort and the pain of a real injury. The ability to distinguish between the two comes with time and experience. It's important to listen to your body, as warning signs usually precede injuries. If you back off and make adjustments at the earliest indication of problems, you'll have a good chance of avoiding forced downtime.

Tendonitis and Bursitis

Tendons are fibrous connective tissues that join muscle to bone. If they become inflamed, the action of pulling the muscle becomes irritating and movement becomes painful. This is called tendonitis or inflammation of the tendon. The same is true for the small sacs of fluid between joints called bursa. Inflammation or irritation of the bursa is called bursitis. Both conditions are often caused by overuse. Symptoms include pain and stiffness in the area aggravated by movement.

Having a good warm-up, correct technique, and a regular stretching program aids in preventing tendonitis and bursitis.

Even with all these precautions, though, some people experience these pains. It happens to the best of us. If it occurs, back off of your training a bit, and be sure to ice the affected area after all workouts.

Plantar Fasciitis and Heel Spurs

The plantar fascia is a band of tissue, much like a tendon, that starts at the heel and runs along the bottom of your foot. It works like a rubber band between the heel and the ball of your foot to form the arch of your foot. Partial tears in this tissue are referred to as plantar fasciitis. Severe tears can cause it to pull away from the heel bone. When this occurs, the bone attempts to heal itself and grows new bone. This excess is referred to as the heel spur and can be very painful.

You can reduce your chance of this injury by maintaining a consistent strength and flexibility program, specifically with attention for your calf muscles. Additionally, choose shoes that have good shock absorption and a supportive arch.

Training Tips

It's good to replace your shoes every 300 to 400 miles. When you buy a new pair, use a permanent marker and write the expiration date somewhere inside them. To determine the expiration date, divide the range of 300 to 400 miles by your weekly running mileage. For example, if you purchased new shoes today and you average 20 miles per week, you should replace them in 15 to 20 weeks.

Iliotibial Band Syndrome

The iliotibial band (ITB), often referred to as the IT band, is a large tendon that runs along the outside of the leg from the knee to the hip. Iliotibial band syndrome is due to excessive friction between the ITB and knee or hip bone, often caused by improper running or biking technique. The result is typically a sharp pain on either side of the knee. It can also cause pain in the hip region (more common in women).

The best way to prevent ITB syndrome is to focus on proper form when running and biking. If you pronate, you should seek adjustments with the right kind of shoe and possibly orthotic inserts. If you run on a track, change directions frequently to help balance out the load and impact on your joints and tendons. Running with a shorter stride also reduces stress to this area. (See Chapter 7 for more efficient running tips.) Proper bike setup can also lower your risks for ITB syndrome, as will a regular stretching routine.

Shin Splints

Shin splints are pains along the tibia or shinbone of the lower leg. The pain runs vertically along the inside or outside of the bone and is often caused from adding too much exercise volume too fast as well as general overuse. Running on hard surfaces such as concrete, tight calf muscles, irregular foot role, and running on crowned (rounded) surfaces can also influence shin splints.

To prevent shin splints, always have a proper warm-up, regularly stretch with a focus on your calf muscles, wear proper footwear (which may include orthotics), and increase mileage gradually.

Chondromalacia Patella (Runner's Knee)

Chondromalacia is due to an irritation of the undersurface of the kneecap (patella). It's covered with a layer of smooth cartilage, which normally glides across the knee as the joint bends. However, in some individuals, the kneecap tends to rub against one side of the knee joint, and the cartilage surface becomes irritated, resulting in knee pain. This can also be caused from overuse.

You can prevent runner's knee by strengthening and stretching out your leg muscles. A good exercise to perform is the leg extension with a focus on the last 15 degrees. (Chapter 10 illustrates the technique for leg extensions.)

Swimmer's Shoulder

Swimmer's shoulder is a condition characterized by soreness and inflammation of the rotator cuff. It's most often caused by the repetitive overhead arm motion of the freestyle stroke.

Swimmer's shoulder can be prevented by performing a 5- to 10-minute warm-up before you get into your main workout. It's also important to use proper freestyle stroke. (We discuss this further in Chapter 5.)

Increases in training distances and frequency should be gradual. If you're too aggressive in your routine, you're likely to wear out your shoulder muscles, leaving them at risk for impingement and shoulder pain. Stretching shoulder, chest, and neck muscles also helps prevent a poor swimming posture. If you think you're at risk, avoid the use of swim paddles and bands, as they increase the load on the shoulder joint.

Training Principles

There are some key guidelines to understand and apply to your training program. They are not exclusive to triathlon, but we will give them a little TRI spin.

Law of *specificity* says that when a specific demand is placed on the body, there will be a specific response. In other words, fitness is specific to a training mode. Swimming makes you become a stronger swimmer. Time spent on the bike makes you a stronger cyclist. Running makes you a stronger runner. We're not saying you shouldn't incorporate other cross-training activities; as we discussed earlier, cross-training has its place. We're just saying, per this principle, that to best prepare yourself for a specific task, you must train specifically.

Coaches' Corner

Steve was chatting with an aerobics and Pilates instructor who works at his local fitness center about swimming. She told him she struggles to swim a full lap (down and back) without stopping. Steve was surprised because she teaches 14 fitness classes a week and she's in excellent shape … but she doesn't ever exercise by swimming. Although she's very fit, her swimming specific muscles and stamina are not ready to perform. To improve in each discipline of TRI, you must spend time in each one.

Law of *overload* says that beneficial adaptations occur in response to demands placed on the body at levels beyond a certain threshold, but within the limits of tolerance. When we train and place stress on our body, it actually becomes temporarily weakened. Then, during the recovery phase, it rebuilds itself stronger than it was originally. It overcompensates and you become slightly more fit. The trick is to stress your body at loads between your threshold and safe limits. Always err on the side of less duration/intensity rather than more. Training is a gradual process. The key is consistency.

Law of *reversibility* says the body's fitness level declines in response to discontinuing a training program. In other words: use it or lose it! When a consistent training streak is broken, the body's condition begins to slip backward. Losses start to be noticeable within 2 to 3 weeks. It's not fair is it? Getting back to where you were before the break takes longer than it does to regress.

Monitoring Yourself

Frequency, *intensity*, and *time* (duration) are blended together in various ways to produce the training schedule and are collectively referred to as *FIT*. Frequency refers to the number of workouts performed in a given timeframe. Intensity is the speed or stress level placed on the body. Time, or duration, is the length of the workout.

We discuss frequency and time in great detail in upcoming chapters when we get into actual training plans and drills. For the time being, we'll focus our attention on intensity.

Understanding Training Intensities

You can measure intensity in several ways, such as VO_2max testing, anaerobic threshold testing, heart-rate formulas, and the rating of perceived exertion (RPE). For our purposes, let's take a look at the latter two—heart rate and RPE. More advanced techniques include graded exercise tests that incorporate many variables such as heart rate, oxygen consumption, lactate levels, and RPE. Some of these specialized tests require specific equipment and should be conducted by an experienced trainer, physician, or exercise physiologist.

Generally speaking, training by heart rate and perceived exertion is easier and often just as accurate when both are used in tandem. Additionally, it saves you a boatload of cash!

Managing Heart-Rate Zones

We break heart rates into four zones. Zone 1 is used early in the training program as well as for active recovery workouts. Zone 2 is great for building aerobic capacity. Zone 3 takes it to the next level; it incorporates aerobic work while it flirts with anaerobic training. Zone 4 is an intense effort at anaerobic threshold. Your fitness level should be at a sufficient capacity before entering zone 4. Always schedule ample recovery following such a workout to allow for effective fitness absorption. Zone 4 is not to be used at the beginning of a training program.

Each zone matches up to the following intensity percentages of maximum heart rate:

♦ *Active recovery, zone 1:* 55 to 65 percent

♦ *Endurance, zone 2:* 65 to 75 percent

♦ *Resistance, zone 3:* 75 to 85 percent

♦ *Threshold, zone 4:* 85 to 90 percent

Use the following formula to calculate your specific zones:

Target heart rate (THR) = (220 – age) × desired intensity percent

For example, zone 3 for a 20-year-old would be:

Lower THR = (220 – 20) × 0.75 = 150

Upper THR = (220 – 20) × 0.85 = 170

The best way to monitor your heart rate zones is by the use of a heart rate monitor, which we mentioned in Chapter 3. The monitor is made up of two main components: a watch and a chest strap. The chest strap detects your heart rate and sends a signal to the watch for real-time readouts. These monitors are becoming the de facto standard when it comes to many cardio-based activities.

The cost of heart-rate monitors depends on the brand and features. Our advice is to get a basic monitor to start with (you can always upgrade later if you decide you'd like to also track elevation, pace, time in Switzerland, etc.). Most allow you to program your intensity levels right into the watch. For example, upon setup, ours asks us to enter our birthday. Based on that data, it calculates our standard zones.

A heart rate monitor makes it easy to be sure you stay in the right intensity zones during training.

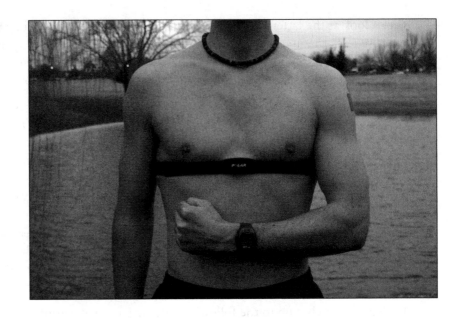

Listen to Your Body

A second method of intensity training is the rate of perceived exertion (RPE). This is more of a "feel" or subjective approach. It was developed by Dr. Gunnar Borg and is also referred to as the Borg Scale. It takes into consideration what you are experiencing and perceiving: psychological, musculoskeletal, and environmental factors as well as overall fatigue. The standard scale ranges from 6 to 20.

Each number carries an associated intensity characterization. For example, 13 (in the middle of the scale) translates to "somewhat hard." Over time, you'll learn how each number correlates to effort. It'll become natural for you to feel what a 13 is, and if your schedule calls for it, maintain the right level of intensity.

Rate of Perceived Exertion

6

7   Very, very light

8

9   Very light

10

11   Fairly light

12

13	Somewhat hard
14	
15	Hard
16	
17	Very hard
18	
19	Very, very hard
20	

> **Training Tips**
>
> Copy the RPE scale and tape it to your wrist or handle bars. This is good to do early on until you learn the association between heart rate and effort.

Borg RPE scale © Gunnar Borg, 1970, 1985, 1994, 1998.

The Right Mixture

Ideally, you'll learn to strike a balance between heart-rate intensities and RPE. This is important because sometimes there's a deviation between the "standard" heart rate and age that would impact the training zones. For example, research has demonstrated that older adults may have significantly higher max heart rates. Women have also been found to generally have higher heart rates at the same levels of work output.

It's best to use the heart-rate formula in combination with the RPE scale. If you find that you have a deviation from the formula, make the adjustments to your training zone numbers. For example, you may find your heart rate is in zone 2 but you only feel you're working in RPE matching moderate output, 12 to 13.

Extreme heat stress and elevation can skew heart rate, too. Both scenarios can result in above-normal heart rates for a given output. RPE is the better indicator in such examples.

Here's a quick breakdown of what your target heart rate and RPE should be for each zone:

◆ *Active recovery, zone 1:* 55 to 65 percent, RPE 12 to 13 (moderate)

◆ *Endurance, zone 2:* 65 to 75 percent, RPE 13 to 15 (somewhat hard)

◆ *Resistance, zone 3:* 75 to 85 percent, RPE 15 to 16 (hard)

◆ *Threshold, zone 4:* 85 to 90 percent, RPE 16 to 18 (very hard)

Ramping It Up

As we mentioned before, the key to TRI training is gradual and consistent exercise. Taking it a "baby step" farther is adding the element of progression. This is just a way of saying you should gradually increase workload (i.e., increase your FIT).

Build the Pyramid

The structure and design of a pyramid provides the perfect example of TRI training. The bottom of it is wide and stout; a solid base. Without a solid foundation, the rest would be impossible. Layers stack together and progress upward toward the peak (a climax). Like the ancient Egyptians, we are building our own pyramids.

The foundation for our pyramid is the *preparation phase*. Depending on the distance of your race/end goal and your personal level of fitness, this can last from 0 to 12 weeks. The prep phase is good for introducing fitness demands to your body, improving technique, and preparing you for the next level. FIT should remain relatively low. You should stay primarily in heart rate zone 1. If you have prior TRI experience or another athletic background, it may be difficult to reign yourself in during this phase. You'll remember back to high-intensity workouts from days of old and want to hammer away. Have patience. You'll thank us later. If you're already working out several times a week and have the skills necessary for TRI, this phase will be very short. If you have never before worked out and feel you need more than 12 weeks to ramp up, go for it. Remember, you are your best coach.

Coaches' Corner

Many discussions about TRI training leave out the prep phase because it's assumed that people have all the skills necessary and some level of fitness before beginning a training program. We believe this is a critical period, especially for those who are just getting into training for the first time (or after a long absence). Remember, you are laying the foundation of your pyramid. Take your time and make it solid.

The first layer in our official training program is the *base phase*. As with a real pyramid, the wider the base of our training pyramid, the higher the peak can be. Therefore, it's important to develop endurance and strength that will carry the weight of future layers. In the base phase, you are still honing and developing skills. Attention to this now pays dividends later. You should keep your heart rate in zones 1 and 2. However, you'll begin to add increments of frequency and duration.

Training Tips

You'll find a greater need for planned and unplanned recovery in the build phase. Always listen to your body!

The next layer of the program is the *build phase*. Sound prep and base periods begin to show their value here. In addition to more intensity and duration, we add key workouts in each discipline. These are priority workouts with a greater focus and should not be missed. Your heart rate should hover primarily between zones 2 and 3. Zone 4 might even come into play during some key workouts.

Our last layer of the pyramid consists of the *peak phase*. Your training duration will begin to decrease, but you'll keep up your frequency. This ensures you don't lose "that loving TRI feeling."

The two main factors of the peak phase are intensity and recovery. Maintain intensity primarily in zones 3 and 4 during key workouts; other workouts should be done at low intensity—zones 1 and 2. This will contribute to your active recovery while allowing you time to focus on tweaking skills and technique.

Toward the end of the peak phase, you will find the *taper*. During the taper, F.I.T. is reduced and recovery becomes the number one priority. The goal is to rid your body of lingering fatigue. This phase typically lasts between 10 and 21 days, depending on your current level of fitness and the race distance. The length of the taper should be longer for a greater-distance triathlon.

Coaches' Corner
Until the tapering segment of the training season, workouts generally get harder and longer. Some athletes have a hard time tapering. They don't want to back off because they feel like they're letting down their guard. The exact opposite is actually true. It takes approximately 10 to 12 days to realize the benefits of a given workout. Therefore, training with a high workload within 10 days of a race reaps no additional fitness benefits. Enjoy the taper!

Take a Look in the Mirror

Just as important as the training principles (laws) of overload, specificity, and reversibility is the law of *individuality*. We all show up with our own DNA genetic code: the number of slow twitch muscle fibers, mitochondria density, fat cell counts and sizes, height, etc. The rate and ability for each of us to improve and grow in the sport somewhat depend on our individuality. This isn't a limitation, just something to take into consideration.

Learn what works for you and make adjustments as necessary. There is no single workout program for everyone. Follow the training principles and guidelines while incorporating your own individuality and you'll get where you need to be.

The Least You Need to Know

- The body has two main energy systems—aerobic (used in endurance events) and anaerobic (used for short bursts of speed/power).

- Avoid injuries by following training principles and guidelines. It's important, too, to listen to your body.

- Monitor your training intensity using your heart rate and RPE.

- Build your TRI training pyramid gradually, progressing through the prep, base, build, and peak phases.

- Take everything you know and learn about TRI conditioning and apply the law of individuality. This is *your* workout. Make it about *you*.

Part 2

You Got Skills, and They're Multiplyin'

Triathlon is composed of three sports: swimming, biking, and running. Almost everyone has taken part, to some extent and at some point in his or her life, in all three sports. As a kid, running is a fundamental part of most outdoor games, and almost all sports involve running to some extent, so we're pretty sure you've done that. Even people who are afraid of the water will get in up to their waist on a hot summer day to cool off. Riding bikes was always a way to experience speed and freedom as a kid, whether you had streamers on the handlebars or a baseball card making noise in the spokes.

Even if you're missing a basis for one or all of these three sports, you'll still be able to achieve in triathlon. To become a triathlete, you just need to be willing to get in the water and start learning or improving your swimming stroke. Give yourself time, and you'll become proficient. You'll have to hop on your bike and start pedaling on a regular basis. Even if your bike is 10 years old with a basket on the front, we make you more efficient in these pages. Running may seem like your arch nemesis now, but we give you a new perspective. For those of you who hated running in gym class, don't worry! We did, too. Running with a purpose and goal is going to change your view of the sport.

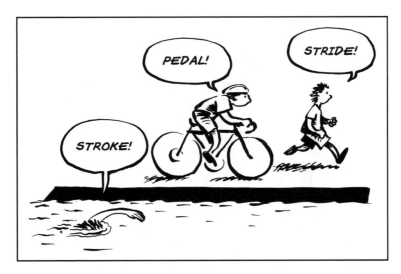

Chapter 5

Have Goggles, Will Swim

In This Chapter

- ◆ Why swimming is so good for you
- ◆ Proper form goes a long way
- ◆ Fun (and smart) swim options
- ◆ Practice drills and workouts

Many people look at swimming as a recreational pastime that goes on at the local pool or on a beach vacation. Most forget that it's one of the best total body workouts you can do. Even in the winter, local fitness clubs or community colleges offer classes and/or open swim times where you can go to stay in shape. Also, because you can choose to do your swimming inside, you don't have to pray for good weather to get in a workout.

Not to mention, splashing around in a big pool of water is still as fun as it was when you were a kid!

The Benefits of Swimming

While it's fun and anyone can learn to do it, swimming also provides some of the greatest fitness benefits, too. Swimming is an "equal opportunity activity." We don't care if you're 8 or 80, if you're a size XXS or XXL, or have two legs or none. We know swimmers who fall in all these categories, and many in each group can lap our butts!

Happy Joints

Not only are there very few possible overuse injuries caused from swimming, but it's often used as part of prescribed injury recovery. Why? You're suspended in a hydro medium (very existential sounding!) that defies gravity. Floating in a pool of water is as close as you can get to the feeling of weightlessness while on our green planet. No other activity on Earth offers such a low degree of impact on the body.

Swimming gives you a great cardio workout while taking it easy on the body. It's a refreshing feeling to come from a workout recharged with happy joints.

Full-Body Activity

Swimming works you inside and out. It's great for your cardio-respiratory systems (heart, lungs), your lower body (legs, hips, glutes), and upper body (core, arms, shoulders). We'd be hard pressed to find any muscle that doesn't fire during a swim workout. Perhaps even the smallest muscle in the body—the middle-ear muscle (stapedius)—gets some work.

Coaches' Corner
Swimming is great for promoting overall body circulation, which is conducive for active recovery sessions. In other words, you can keep aerobic conditioning volumes high without compromising recovery from bike and run training. The nature of swimming enables you to keep developing your cardio fitness while at the same time promoting recovery from your other training. What a kicker!

Technically Speaking

Trust us, technique is the key when swimming. It's more important than size, shape, strength, and even conditioning. Given that water is 1,000 times denser than air, your inefficiencies are magnified greatly if your form is even slightly off. Swimming with poor technique is like swimming against the current. Efficiency in the water pays serious dividends during the bike and run segments of triathlon.

Before we get into the technique aspects, let's drill down into what goes into a basic freestyle stroke:

1. *Hand entry:* Slice your hand in like a knife (approximately 8 to 12 inches in front of your head). Stab the water, make an imaginary hole in the surface of the water, and follow your hand with the rest of your arm. Angle your hand with your palm facing inward, and lead with your little finger (like a slow-mo karate chop).

2. *Catch:* Slightly pause with your extended hand as it catches/gets traction on the water.

3. *Pull:* Pull your hand backward along your side toward your feet, and press the water back by extending your arm to approximately 90 percent of its full extension. Be sure to keep it in line with your body to contribute to good hydrodynamics. Your arm is now ready for the recovery elbow first.

4. *Recovery:* Your opposite side elbow leaves the water, with your elbow high and your hand relaxed directly under it. Your fingers trail on/near the water and then reach forward to the entry position.

A good stroke consists of reaching long, following your hand into the water, a slight pause, and then pulling the water back along your side. Be sure to keep the pull along your side. Imagine that you have two rails on either side of you to guide your arms.

Find Your Buoy: Chest Down, Butt Up

Steve learned to swim "old school." He was taught, like many, to swim free style facing forward, head out of the water, with windmill arms. He was at practically a 45-degree angle! That's not what you want to do, as that creates an uphill battle.

Finding your buoy is about finding float and balance. You want your body to be as horizontal in the water as possible. One way to do this is to relax in the water. The first step is to swim with your head in the water, facing toward the bottom of the pool. Next, press with your chest. In other words, press down between your arm pits. Push your body toward the bottom of the pool. When you do these two things, your bottom half will rise. It's all about finding balance in the water. When you find it, you'll be close to horizontal and that much closer to efficient swim mechanics.

> **Coaches' Corner**
>
> It's important that you bond with the water; feel comfortable and confident that you'll be all right. If you need to spend some time just floating, holding your breath under water, or splashing around—do it. Be one with the water, and you'll be on your way.

Reach for It

When you're swimming, you have to think *l-o-n-g*. Make yourself as tall as possible in the water. The greater the distance between your fingertips and your toes, the better.

When you swim, imagine you're reaching for the edge of a horizontal wall with one hand. When you're fully extended, pause, and then pull yourself over it. Maximizing your reach helps you go farther with each stroke.

Focus on reducing the number of strokes you take per lap. For example, if it takes you 18 strokes to cross the pool, try to exaggerate the length of each stroke until you can gradually reduce the stroke count to below 18. You can use it as a guage to track progress. Comparing your count from workout to workout adds motivation as you watch the number of strokes go down.

def•i•ni•tion

Swimming velocity (SV) equals how far you travel on each stroke (stroke length; SL) times how fast you take each stroke (stroke rate; SR): $SV = SL \times SR$.

The idea is to find the right *swimming velocity* (*SV*), or balance between your stroke length (SL) and your stroke rate (SR) or cadence. It's more efficient to swim with focus on SL. Faster stroke rate does not necessarily mean you'll have a higher *velocity*. Spinning your wheels is a sure way to waste energy. It's important to find the sweet spot between SL and SR. Just never sacrifice the length of each stroke for a higher stroke rate, as the latter is more energy expensive!

Swim on Your Side

Swimming horizontal and swimming long both contribute to improving your hydrodynamics. The final piece is swimming on your side. We know this might sound confusing, as we just talked about being horizontal. The goal is to move away from swimming flat. Colin learned to swim semi–old school. He was taught to swim head down, horizontal, but flat. When we say *flat* we mean chest square and facing toward the bottom of the pool. Swimming like this creates *drag*. Swimming on your side significantly reduces this resistance.

def•i•ni•tion

Drag is the force from turbulence of water against the body. Swimming horizontal, long, and on your side all contribute to reducing drag. You can reduce the impeding force by up to 70 percent by following these principles. Getting from A to B becomes easier, faster, and more fun.

Imagine reaching out with your left arm (beginning your stroke). Now we're going to add a roll into the mix. The roll begins with your core/hips. Reaching with your left arm, you're going to roll to the left side of your body while you pull the water back along your right side. It's like gliding on your side for a second. Then your core/hips will rotate you to the other side. Now you're reaching out with your right arm, rolling to the right side of your body and pulling the water back along your left. You're essentially gliding on each side linked by the quick rolls. You can exaggerate this movement by aiming your belly button at the sides of the pool when you roll.

It might take some time to get used to swimming on your side, but once you get comfortable there, you'll notice how effective this position can be.

Inhale: Left, Right, Left

Before we get into the next principle of swimming, let's take a look at basic breathing technique. It is one of, if not the most critical, elements of swimming. When you have an efficient ability to exchange oxygen and carbon dioxide, you'll be more comfortable in the water, and as a result, better able to focus on other swimming dynamics.

In swim breathing, the exhalation occurs with a forceful blowing through the mouth. It's best if you exhale underwater as you stroke. However, if that doesn't come easy to you, you can also exhale above the water. Just keep in mind that you have limited time. When exhalation is complete, you inhale by turning your head just slightly at the top of your body rotation and sucking in all the air you can get during this brief moment when your face is out of the water. This movement of the head should be as subtle as possible. Think of it as more of a head pivot or swivel.

When Steve first had someone look at his form, he learned that he swam in a curve or at an angle. It became especially noticeable when he did a couple triathlons and swam off course, adding yardage and wasting energy and time. He strayed off track partly because he only took breaths only from his right side. Breathing only to one side can limit your perception of where you are in relation to everything else. It can also contribute to steering you off in an angle. When he started practicing *bilateral breathing*, his swim straightened out.

Training Tips

Practice stealth: during your laps, listen to yourself moving through the water. Focus on the noise you're making. Generally speaking, the quieter you are, the better. If you're thrashing around, it's likely that you're creating turbulence. Paying attention to sound can provide you with a warning sign to refocus on your mechanics.

def•i•ni•tion

Bilateral breathing is simply alternating breaths between your left and right sides. We like to switch on the three-stroke count: left, right, left, *breathe*; right, left, right, *breathe*; etc. However, you can change it up on the fly when you're in need of air or establish your own pattern. This type of breathing is a little more difficult than breathing to one side, but anyone at any level can learn the technique. It just takes some getting used to.

When you master breathing on both sides, you'll feel more confident in the water. It's especially handy when you're in a triathlon surrounded by other competitors. You'll see the action on both sides of you instead of just one, improving your awareness and direction.

Additionally, this ability is extremely helpful anytime there's swell or waves hitting you from one side. You can just breathe to one side, away from the waves. Having the ability to alternate sides can be priceless in many situations.

To Kick or Not to Kick?

Many people think you have to kick like crazy to keep moving forward, but this is a misconception. Most triathletes do very little swimming with their legs. When you learn to apply the techniques we outlined earlier in this chapter, you won't need to spend much energy kicking. It's very energy intensive to keep those large leg muscles moving, with small returns, especially when you'll want to save some juice for the bike and the run.

Coaches' Corner
An easy experiment will prove the truth of kicking: next time you're in the water, time how long it takes you to kick across the pool without using your arms. Then, use a pull buoy or kickboard to keep your legs afloat and time yourself using just your arms. Unless you're part dolphin, we're betting you'll be more than twice as fast when you use your arms.

Training Tips

A good place to increase your kick cadence in a triathlon is toward the end of the swim segment. This increases blood flow to your legs and helps prepare them for the transition and bike portions of the race.

We are not saying not to kick; we're saying it should be secondary. Some swimmers have a natural and efficient ability to kick in conjunction with their overall swim rhythm. That's great. Steve had an awkward kick with inflexible ankles, so it made more sense for him to focus on body roll, stroke length, balance, etc. However, kicking is good for learning and maintaining balance in the water. Your legs serve almost like one of those long poles tightrope walkers use to balance while they walk the tightrope. They help counter balance the body between strokes, pulls, and rolls. (We look more at kicking in the later drills sections.)

Where Can I Swim?

Depending on where you live, the possibilities of where to swim may vary. If you live in a cold climate, you might not have any outdoor pools or open water available year round, so your swim workouts might be limited to laps at the indoor pool. If you're lucky enough to live in a warm climate, you might have the opportunity to swim in outdoor pools and/or in lakes, rivers, or the ocean.

The same techniques can be practiced in any body of water; however, those who have access to a variety of options may obtain a more well rounded experience level. Swim in as many different environments as possible. If your goal race is going to be an outdoor one, we strongly recommend that you practice swimming at least a couple times in open water. You don't want to show up at your first race in a lake/ocean having never experienced what it's like to face a beach start with oncoming waves.

Depending on where you live, you might need to really get bundled up for an outdoor swim.

(Photo by Lois Schwartz)

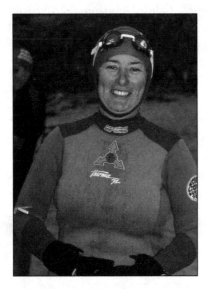

Coming to a Pool Near You ...

Pools are great places to practice and learn proper technique. You don't need to worry about current, waves, or visibility. You can follow the black line and focus on your form. Just be sure you don't have the "death by laps" mind-set: it's not how much time you log in the pool; it's the quality of that time that counts. If you're swimming 3,000 yards a day but maintaining poor technique, your efficiency and speed will remain near the same. Steve's old football coach used to say, "Practice does not make perfect. Rather, perfect practice makes perfect."

Be sure to follow pool etiquette. Some of the rules are common sense, and some are not. Consider the following next time you're going for a swim:

- No diving; slide in or take the steps.

- If you're in a lane with someone else, you can split it or ask if they'd rather circle the lane.

- If you're circling in the lane, it's usually done in a counterclockwise direction (e.g., swim down the right side of the lane, turn at the wall, and swim back on the opposite side).

> **Gravel Ahead**
>
> Be sure to wear waterproof or water-repellant sunscreen if you're swimming outside. Keep a bottle of spray or lotion in your swim bag at all times. Every study published seems to recommend an SPF 30 or above. Remember to reapply as frequently as stated on the bottle (at a minimum).

- If you need to pass, tap the foot ahead of you once or twice to give a signal. After you hit the next wall, pass on the left.

- If you need rest, squeeze into the right corner and let others swim past you.

- Don't block any clocks swimmers might be using to track their pace/intervals.

You have two main options when it comes to pool swimming: swim laps on your own or you can find a Masters' program. If possible, we recommend incorporating both into your schedule. Lap swimming is good when you're practicing drills or your own specific training workout. Lap swim times are usually flexible, and most pools have several options throughout the day. Masters' programs are great because they're coached and goal specific. Typically, the lanes are divided by skill level. For example, lane 1 is the slowest (novice) lane, 2 is a step faster, and 6 is the fastest (advanced) lane. The order may be reversed.

Open-Water Swims

Open water is great for adding variety and challenge to your swim training. Whether it's in a lake, river, or an ocean, you get a whole new experience. There's no line to follow, no wall to grab, and no lane dividers. At first this can be downright scary. It's okay. Hang in there. The more time you spend in open water, the more relaxed you'll become.

When swimming in open water, keep a couple techniques beyond the standard ones in mind.

Raise your elbows a little higher than normal. This is necessary due to waves, swells, or any increase in the water's wake. Obviously, this is not an issue in the pool. Raising your elbows during the stroke helps prevent you from getting thrown off balance.

Training Tips

Wearing a wetsuit helps keep you warm and increases overall buoyancy (lightness in the water). With these two advantages, you can definitely improve your swim times.

Lift your head out of the water and look forward (instead of to the side) from time to time to "sight." Without the black line you're used to at the bottom of the pool, you need to look for buoys, lifeguard towers, or any sort of landmark you can use to check your position while you're on the move. Even if you decide you're going to just follow the feet of another swimmer directly in front of you, you should still sight every once in a while to be sure you're not being led astray.

Safety Check

Always, always, *always* use the buddy system when swimming in open water (or swimming at a pool without a lifeguard). Swim with at least one partner at all times. Also be sure you heed surf reports (check online, in newspapers, and on TV) and lifeguard warnings. Typically, you'll see a hazard flag flying under dangerous conditions. It's best to avoid swimming during these times.

When you go out and there's a lifeguard station, enter the water in front of the station. Be sure the lifeguard(s) see you go out. That way they'll know to keep an eye on you.

If you find yourself swimming in a strong current or riptide, don't panic. Stay calm and swim parallel to the shore until it subsides and then head back in. Don't attempt to fight the current head on. Taking the angled approach is much easier and safer.

And when you swim off shore, be mindful of how far out you go. It's better to stay in closer and swim parallel to the shore than to swim directly out into the sea for half the time/distance you want to swim. That way, you can get back to land quickly if need be.

Get to Work: Swimming!

Drills are great for learning how to swim, improving your technique, or relearning to swim. Each one builds upon the other until you have the finished product—efficient swimming. Breaking swimming down into manageable chunks is the best way to improve. When you learn one chunk, you can move on to the next. Before you know it, you'll be leading your lane at a Master's swim program!

Water Comfort Basics

Before we get too wet, let's start with the basics. It's important to relax in the water; you need to feel comfortable. For some people, this is not an issue. However, for others, it may take some time. Try rolling on your back and floating. Spend some time underwater holding your breath. While holding onto the wall of the pool, practice bouncing up and down in the water (also known as "bobs"). This may seem very elementary, but for those who are new to swimming, it's good practice. Becoming comfortable in the water can be half the battle for many triathletes.

One of the major challenges we face in swimming is overcoming oxygen debt and managing carbon dioxide levels. Swimming and drills contribute to improving your body's ability to deal with lower oxygen/higher CO_2 levels. Over time, your tolerance will develop, and as a result, you'll feel more comfortable in the water.

Gravel Ahead

Be careful when using swimming aids such as pull buoys, fins, paddles, kickboards, etc. Many times these only temporarily mask poor swim mechanics. They provide a punch when you use them, but it disappears when you put them down. Use them in moderation, and avoid becoming dependent.

Drill One: Chest Down, Butt Up

One of your major technique goals is to keep your legs from dragging as you swim. When your head is high and your butt and legs are low, you're really hurting your hydrodynamics. "Chest down, butt up" will help you be conscious of this.

Starting at the edge of the pool, push off with your face down and your arms to your sides. Use your core muscles to push your chest down and let your hips lift. The objective is to become horizontal with the surface of the water. You don't have to force it by using your leg or back muscles. The physics will take over.

When you find balance, gently kick to move yourself forward. Your head is down and only lifts for air. Notice how your lower half drops when your head surfaces. When you put it back down, you'll regain balance.

Training Tips

If, in any of these balancing drills, your kick doesn't propel you well enough, throw on some fins. They are a good tool when you're learning balance.

Drill Two: Back Down, Butt Up

Next we'll work on learning balance from a 180-degree rotation. Take drill one and reverse it. Face up with your arms to your sides. Push down through your shoulder blades. You're simulating the same balancing technique as in drill one. Gently kick yourself across the pool. Be careful not to hit your head when you approach the wall. You might want to keep an arm out as you get close to it.

Drill Three: Body Roll

Now let's combine drills one and two. Start face down (head in line with your spine), arms at your sides, kicking gently. When you need air, roll onto your back. All the while, maintain balance and originate the roll with your hips so your hips, head, and body all roll together at the same time. This establishes consistent balance. Think about it as though you are swinging a baseball bat. The swing originates with your hips. The energy then rolls from there.

On your back, catch your breath, and roll back to your stomach. Continue doing laps in this fashion. Alternate clockwise to counterclockwise rolls.

Drill Four: Tall Buoy

This drill takes "butt up" and adds extended arms, teaching balance in a different way by adding the element of length into the equation. Face down, arms out in front, kick gently across the pool. Turn your head for air. If your form suffers a little but you can breathe, we think that's a fair trade-off. As you practice more and more with this drill, try to keep your form strong while also being able to breathe.

Drill Five: Sideways

Push off the wall on your side with your lower arm extended out in front and the other to your side, and kick gently. Keep your face pointed toward the bottom of the pool with your cheek against your bicep. Point your belly button at the side of the pool wall. When you need air, turn your head until your mouth is above the water line and take a breath. If you had a straight line running through your hips or shoulder blades, you'd want this line to hit the pool bottom directly underneath where you're swimming.

Initially, most people will be rolled too far on their back or belly instead of exactly sideways in the water. Although it will be hard to strike the perfect balance at first, this drill will really help with efficiency when we put it all together. Alternate sides after each pool length.

Drill Six: Tall Buoy, with Stroke

Incorporating all the previous drills, we'll start to stroke with your arms, one at a time. Before one arm is able to start its stroke, you're going to wait for the first to "catch up" and touch it.

Push off the wall with your face down, arms extended, on your belly, kicking gently. When you need air, take a stroke and breathe at the same time. Then alternate sides. For example, you're kicking along with both arms extended: pull your right arm along your side, and when it gets near your hip, roll onto your left side. Roll your head with your hips, take a breath, and return to the starting point (catch-up position). Then alternate sides—stroking and breathing.

Training Tips

You're in the water for a swim workout, so you obviously don't feel yourself sweating, but trust us, you are! Swimming burns approximately 3 calories a mile per pound of bodyweight. If you weigh 160 pounds and it takes you 30 minutes to swim a mile, you burn about 960 calories in an hour if your pace remains constant. Bring a bottle of water or sports drink with you to your next swim workout so you're sure to stay hydrated, and have a post-workout snack ready to go.

Drill Seven: Three-Count Stroke

Next let's speed things up a bit. You're still rolling and alternating sides, but now you increase the turn over. Start on one of your sides with your bottom arm extended. After a "3 count," complete half a stroke with your top arm while rolling to the center (both arms extended). Hold this position for 3 seconds. Complete half a stroke with the opposite arm and roll onto the other side for 3 seconds. Repeat. Remember to keep your balance and roll head and hips together. Breathe as needed. Now you're starting to establish the swimming vibe.

Drill Eight: Touch Catch-Up

Now you're going to start on one side, stroke, touch the other hand in front, pause, and pull through to the other side. Essentially, you're swimming normally with a pause out front. The catch-up gives you a reference point to return to after each stroke. Your body is rolling, and you're reaching long and pulling next to your side.

Keep practicing each drill in progression. When you feel you've learned one, advance to the next. When you're confident with all eight drills, shift your goal to fine-tuning your mechanics and learning precise timing. Your objective is to maximize the force that goes into each stroke. In other words, you want the biggest bang for your buck. You'll learn how to keep momentum between strokes. In doing this, you'll become aware of traction. When there's a good rhythm in your overall swim mechanics, your hands will move at the same rate as your body. You'll limit what is called slipping; which simply means that your hands are moving as they stroke, but you don't feel like you're getting anywhere. Remember, efficient swimming is about long glides linked by quick rolls.

Training Tips

If you're swimming in a crowd (in a pool or open water), you might be able to draft off another swimmer. By positioning yourself right behind someone and letting them cut the water. Staying near their feet gives you the benefit of reduced turbulence by falling in behind their wake. Some refer to it as a "free ride." It's not exactly free, but it does help. Find someone who swims at your pace or just a fuzz faster. It saves energy, and it's 100 percent legal.

Swimming Review

Swimming is like golf; a lot of little things go into good results. Here's a mental checklist to keep in mind:

❑ Press down with your chest (balance).

❑ Keep your head down (in line with your spine) and get air when you're in the turn.

❑ Originate rolls with your hips (core).

❑ Head, shoulders, trunk, and hips all roll together.

❑ Reach long and swim on your sides.

❑ Don't cross over the centerline of your body during your strokes.

❑ Keep your hands along your side during the pull. (Imagine there's a box around you and stay within it.)

❑ During the pull, focus on pulling the water back along your side. This helps propel you forward.

❑ Leave one arm out in front when the other is pulling. (This keeps you long at all times.)

Here's a list of swim talk that will help prepare you for your workouts:

intervals   Specific distances performed within a specific duration, e.g., 50 yards on 0:55 (55 seconds).

pace   How fast you're swimming a specific distance, e.g., 100 yards in 1:30 (minute and a half).

pace clock   A large clock displayed on the deck of a pool; use the clock to track both how fast you're swimming as well as rest time.

repeats   A repetition of the distance you swim within each interval; they usually range from 25 to 800 yards.

rest   Time taken after each interval.

set   A series of intervals/repeats, e.g., 4 × 100 yards is a set in which you swim 100-yard intervals, 4 times in a row.

So let's review. What does the following example mean?

Set: 3 × 100 yards on 2:15

This means you're swimming 100 yards on the 2-minute, 15-second interval. After you finish your first 100, you'll rest until 2:15 has elapsed and then head out for your second. Repeat until you've finished the set.

Sample Workouts

Swim workouts should include a warm-up, sets (with designated intervals), and a cool-down:

Warm-up: Swim an easy 10 minutes to gradually elevate your heart rate and get your blood flowing. You can mix in different strokes such as freestyle, breaststroke, backstroke, etc.

Set(s): Swim a distance/interval, repeat, and apply duration and rest periods. Sets have a purpose, such as to develop skills, endurance, speed, muscular endurance, or anaerobic conditioning. You can have multiple sets within a given workout.

Cool-down: Swim an easy 10 minutes to get your heart rate down and even out your body's stress hormones.

> ### Coaches' Corner
> If you ever hear the phrase "choice of stroke," you can choose whichever you'd like. If there's no indication of a particular stroke, the freestyle is usually the default.

We get into more suggestions for planning workouts in Chapter 12.

The Least You Need to Know

◆ Swimming is a full-body activity anyone can do.

◆ Proper swimming technique is more important than physical condition.

◆ Bilateral breathing increases spatial awareness and improves swimming direction.

◆ Practice safety: swim with a partner when in open water or in pools without lifeguards.

◆ Drill progression should be from most basic to most complex.

Chapter 6

Let's Ride Bikes!

In This Chapter

- ◆ Maximizing efficiency on the bike
- ◆ Learning some minor mechanics
- ◆ Smart, safe, and fun riding options
- ◆ Workout ideas

As a kid, your bike was a way to get around without having to rely on your parents. It meant freedom. It meant exploration. It still does. Your bike is a great way to both exercise and get from point A to point B. Once you start, you won't be able to stop. Pedal on ….

The Benefits of Cycling

Some of the first bikes date back to the mid-1800s. Although the styles, geometries, and qualities have changed significantly over the years, some things remain the same. Bikes are simple means of transportation, recreation, and fun. The underlying benefits of each involve an elevated quality of health. You bike for fitness. You bike for stress-relief. You bike to feel like a kid again.

Cycling: A Low-Impact Sport

Compared with running, the bike rates really well on the low-impact-activity index (swimming is still less impact). Your upper body virtually takes on no load except for supporting its own weight. By using aero bars, you can even transfer some weight from a muscle-bearing to a skeletal-bearing load (i.e., your bones will support your upper body with almost no energy expended). The lower body takes on some force through the ankles, knees, and hips; however, good form can help reduce overall impact. Generally speaking, biking is safe for people of all ages and fitness levels.

Strengthen Those Legs

Ideally, when you cycle, you want to have a "quiet" upper body. This just means it shouldn't move much. Keep things up top still and relaxed. Your upper body should be used for balance, steering, and to grab your water bottle when necessary. Let your legs and lower body handle the work.

Some people think the quadriceps or thighs handle most of the effort, but in reality, when practicing good form, you work your quadriceps, hamstrings, calves, and the strongest muscle in the body—the gluteus maximus, a.k.a. the butt.

The type of terrain you ride on affects how your cycling legs develop. If you ride hills, you'll build stronger legs more quickly than you would from riding on level ground. You'll work harder to get up the hills but then get a respite on your way down. Riding on more level ground, or flats, also has its challenges. You'll use fewer muscle groups, but the ones that do fire can get overworked. On the flats, you'll probably keep a constant pace at all times with little opportunity to coast and take a break.

Anywhere you ride has its own challenges and stresses your legs in different ways, both for training rides and races. We recommend riding on all types of terrains if you live in an area where this is possible.

> **Training Tips**
>
> Training in several topographies conditions your leg muscles in a comprehensive manner. All riding builds strength; however, when you mix up the terrain, your muscles get more well-rounded workouts.

Try to train on roads that resemble the course of the triathlon race you're preparing for. If the race will be held in a land far, far away, you might be able to find out what sort of course you'll encounter by looking it up online. If you can't find anything on the web, contact the race director to try to get a feel for the course. When you figure out what the course is going to be like, if possible, you should try to be sure at least some of your training rides are on similar terrain.

Technically Speaking

The bike segment is sandwiched between the swim and the run parts of the triathlon. When you get off the bike, you'll need to have energy left over to conquer the run. One way to be sure this happens is to maintain good technique. Proper form reduces the amount of energy needed, as less wasted energy on the bike means more energy for the run. This is your goal.

The importance of good technique may seem more obvious to you in swimming, because biking, for many, is second nature. You just have to pedal, right? Not exactly.

Pedal Faster (Physics of Cadence)

Remember our conversation about lactic acid in Chapter 4? Lactate is your body's buffering agent for the acid that builds up in your muscles during exercise. When the acid level rises faster than your body can process it, you feel a burning sensation in your muscles. When you're riding in a harder gear, your pedal strokes are slower and the acid can build up very fast. At the other end of the spectrum, if you are in a lower gear and there's little resistance, you may have a very fast pedal stroke. You want to find that sweet spot between power and endurance. You want to find the perfect pedaling rhythm … tempo … cadence.

Everything has a cadence. You breathe with a cadence. Your heart beats at a cadence. You'll ride at one, too. In cycling terminology, cadence is best understood when looking at revolutions per minute (RPM). How many times do your pedals go around in 1 minute? Generally speaking, on flat ground, the optimal range is between 80 and 100. Riding down hills may raise your cadence while riding up hills will probably bring it down (although shifting gears will compensate for some of that).

Gravel Ahead

You don't want to train at too high or too low a cadence. Either extreme will cause your legs to fatigue more quickly than necessary. Monitor your cadence to keep it between 80 and 100, either using a bike computer or manually. You can easily figure out your cadence while riding by counting the number of times your right knee rises in 10 seconds and multiplying by 6. This gives you your RPM or cadence.

To achieve the ideal cadence range, you must shift gears. Most riders of all levels do not shift enough, which leads to inconsistent cadence and effort. Shift, shift, shift. It takes time and practice to learn the gears, find your RPM range, and maintain desired intensity zones. A bike computer can assist you by tracking such things as cadence, speed, miles covered, and time elapsed. When we ride, we pay most attention to our cadence in conjunction with intensity.

Good Form

When you were a kid, your bike probably had standard, flat pedals. You just pushed the pedals down; first on the one side and then the other. The mind-set was all about that down motion. Your goal now is to get away from that way of thinking. Earlier we talked about how cycling should trigger many muscles of the lower body. If you were to simply push down, you'd greatly limit total muscle involvement, which would lead to faster muscle fatigue.

Good form on the bike centers around the "full circle" mentality. The goal is to make your leg muscles spin your foot and the pedal in little circles. Physically, this obviously happens just by making the pedal go around.

Coaches' Corner

We highly recommend upgrading your pedals so you can at least somewhat secure your feet. Consider investing in some pedal straps or clipless pedals.

However, we want you to focus on making each foot go around in tiny circles. You shouldn't just be pushing down with one leg and then waiting for the next time that same leg can push down. For more efficiency and power, you should be exerting force in nearly all 360 degrees as the pedal makes its rotation.

Think finesse. Think smooth. Think circular. If you push forward (imagine pushing your toes out through your shoes), the down stroke comes naturally because you've been doing it for years. Then focus on pulling backward (image sliding your heel back through your shoe) and through the 7, 8, and 9 of a clock face. This pedal stroke moves away from the up and down mentality and incorporates the forward, backward, and up movements—hence the "full circle" mind-set. The result is a much more efficient spin. You'll post better numbers with less energy.

The other spot where some cyclists can improve their efficiency is their "line." Your line is the path your bike takes on the road. Keeping your front tire pointed directly ahead in the direction you're going seems obvious, but many riders constantly make tiny corrections that cause their bikes to swerve back and forth very slightly on the road. Every time the bike is not going directly straight, the distance the tires are covering is increased slightly.

Don't ride over potholes and shiny objects just to keep a good line, but when the road ahead is clear, keep your focus a bit ahead of you to avoid too many overcorrections—just like you do when driving a car.

Coaches' Corner

Aero bars have only been around since 1989 and offer cyclists a way to "cheat the wind." Aero bars take some getting used to at first, so practice getting into and out of the aero position in low-traffic areas when no one is in front of you. The position will feel somewhat awkward at first because it changes how your weight is distributed (there's a shift forward in weight and balance). Also, you won't have your brakes at your fingertips, so only get aero when you're comfortable with the road ahead, traffic, etc. When you're comfortable with aero, you'll have better aerodynamics and less load on your upper body's muscular system. Just use discretion for when you decide to get aero.

Going the Distance (Pacing)

The pace at which you ride depends on the purpose and duration of the ride. If it's an easy training day, your pace might be slower than normal. If you're racing in a sprint-distance triathlon, your pace may be near maximum effort. If you're competing in an Ironman-distance TRI, your pace may be moderate and consistent. If you're training in an interval group bike class, your pace may vary from easy to intense.

Pacing is an important component of the bike discipline and can be difficult to master at first. Know yourself, your goals, and your race. It's easy to get caught up in what someone else is doing and fall out of your zones. When this happens, refocus on your RPM, intensity, and overall status. Make adjustments as necessary, but find your groove. Over time and with experience, pacing becomes more second nature.

Where Should I Ride?

You can ride anywhere you feel comfortable, on any terrain your bike can handle. For most of us, this means sticking to the streets and paved bike paths. For those with a mountain bike, feel free to spice things up with some trail riding. Just remember, always stay in control and keep it safe!

Low-Traffic Streets and Paths

No matter what kind of bike you're on, safety is the first priority when riding. (We cover more road safety tips in the later "Safety Check" section.) Generally, the less traffic, the better the area is to bike. Even if every person behind the wheel of every vehicle on the road were a great driver, the size and speed of the vehicles should still make them a serious consideration. A bike will never win a bike-versus-car collision. If someone is eating behind the wheel and drops a french fry or if their cell phone rings, they might take their eyes off the road and start to veer toward you. Find the safest roads you can, but be aware that you're taking a calculated risk anytime you're out on a public road.

Training Tips

When you're riding on the road, take a quick glance over your left shoulder from time to time. If on a low-traffic street, you notice a car and you're riding with a partner yell out "Car back," to keep everyone informed.

It helps to know the area before heading out. Get a map if you have to, and look for routes off the beaten path. As poet Robert Frost said, "take the road less traveled."

Some cities have bike lanes on certain roads. If you're lucky enough to have these specific lanes for you to travel in, take advantage of them. The space the lane provides should help buffer you from other traffic. You still need to be vigilant in your travels, though; vehicles might not be paying attention, and a white line on the road is not a true barrier.

You also might be able to find bike paths in your area. These are typically located in a park or forest preserve and are shut off from most vehicular traffic. Bike paths give you a break from worrying about traffic and stop signs or stoplights. You can just ride, focusing on your form and pace. Generally, you stay to your right, as oncoming cyclists may approach on your left. When you approach another rider or runner and want to pass, call out "Passing on your left."

Training Tips

When you're riding in front of other riders and notice there's something on the road to avoid, give signals. You can point in the direction of the hazard prior to avoiding it. This gives the other riders behind you a heads-up.

Be aware that some of these paths have speed limits. Although they may have never applied to you before, they may be a consideration now that you're in training. We've never heard of anyone being "pulled over" for speeding on a bike path, but there are firsts for everything so be sure you abide by the rules of the path.

For more on sharing the road with automobiles and other road safety, check out the "Safety Check" section later in this chapter.

Hills? Wind? Bring It On!

When you're comfortable riding on flat and rolling terrain, you might want to challenge yourself with some climbing and/or other more difficult rides. Steeper hills help improve muscular strength and endurance and give you an opportunity to stand up from time to time, recruit more muscle groups, and stretch out a little. In addition to the physical benefits of climbing, you'll also appreciate the change of scenery. If you don't live in the mountains, going for a hill workout might take you to new places with amazing landscapes.

> ### Coaches' Corner
>
> Whenever Colin goes for a ride in the hills, he takes his digital camera (enclosed in a resealable plastic bag to protect it from sweat) in his jersey pocket for any picturesque scenes. Look out, Ansel Adams!

Riding into a strong headwind or with a crosswind will make your ride harder, but it definitely will benefit you during training. You don't want to find yourself in a triathlon with a fierce crosswind if you've never been in the situation before. Learning how to handle your bike during crazy-strong winds in training is priceless. When this happens, stay calm and do your best to stay "in your line."

Facing a strong headwind is less about danger and more about spirit. Your form might be good and your effort consistent, but with a strong headwind, the results you want won't be there. It can be downright depressing. Stay strong. If this happens to you during training, you'll get a great workout. If it happens during a race, remember that the other athletes are suffering along with you. Everyone's time will be slower.

 Training Tips

If you're facing a mighty headwind, get aero. If you have a set of aero bars on your bike, use them. If not, lower yourself into the drops (the lower part of the handlebars on a standard "10 speed"). From sitting up, to the drops, to aero bars, you'll reduce the amount of body area facing directly into the wind. Get low and give the wind less to push on!

Indoor Options

Those of us who live in areas that aren't conducive to outdoor riding must head inside. Indoor options are also good if you need a break from outside worries such as traffic, potholes, weather, etc., or if you want to do a specific timed workout in a controlled environment. Some popular indoor choices include stationary bikes, turbo-trainers, and group classes.

Stationary bikes you find at most fitness centers are good if you're in a pinch or traveling without your bike. These machines can get your heart rate up just like your regular bike, but they have limited adjustability and they usually don't have similar geometries as your personal bike. Cycling on a bike with a drastically different setup can lead to injury, so try to avoid them if possible.

Turbo-trainers (or bike trainers) are great because you can set them up with your own bike. These devices maintain consistent biomechanics with your regular outdoor riding. (Biomechanics is a fancy way of saying that both internal and external forces impact your body depending on one's position, technique, and overall movement.) Trainers range from simple to complex. Some just elevate your back wheel, add resistance, and enable you to spin indoors. Others have tons of bells and whistles such as computer readout information (watts, speed, cadence, etc.) and video imagery hookups (scenery programs or other readouts). We both have the former and like to keep these workouts relatively simple. We set up our bikes in front of the TV and spin to a good movie or sitcoms on the DVR.

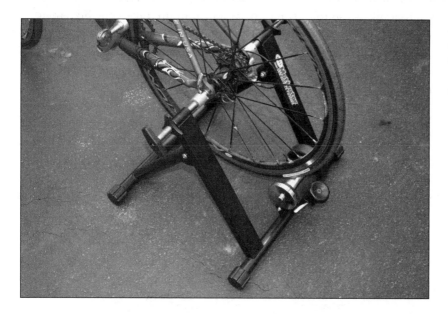

Bike trainers enable you to have a focused bike workout in a controlled environment (and are also great for bad-weather days).

Coaches' Corner

Generally speaking, your indoor cycling options often offer a greater minute-for-minute value than an outdoor ride because you're always spinning. You can't coast along with the wind at your back for a little break. Inside, if you stop cranking, the wheels stop spinning. There's an estimated time-and-a-half advantage, too: if you get a good 1-hour spin in, it's worth roughly an hour and a half of your average road ride. Don't think you should condense all your bike workouts by getting them done on a trainer. Just be aware so that when you do take it indoors, if your workout is a little shorter, you're still getting in a great workout.

Joining a group exercise class like Spinning can add both extra motivation and a social aspect to your bike workouts. The classes are lead by an instructor, and each session has a specific goal. For example, the ride might focus on endurance or intervals. As with most of the workouts we discuss, these classes usually involve a warm-up, workout, and cool-down followed by stretching. Sessions usually last about 60 minutes, and after the class, you'll feel like it was a very efficient time spent improving your cardio fitness and overall bike conditioning.

Bike Mechanic 101

When you own a bike, it's going to need some TLC from time to time. You might have to take it apart for traveling, oil the chain, change a flat tire, etc. You should take some time to learn to do these things on your own. When you pick up these skills, you'll save time, money, and possible frustration down the road (and on the road).

Even if you do perform basic maintenance on your two-wheeled steed, every once in a while you should try to get it into a bike shop for a tune-up. At a minimum, take your bike in at the beginning of the season. You might consider taking it in again a week or so before a big race. Just be sure to make an appointment and know when they'll be able to get it back to you. You don't want to miss an important workout because you were waiting for the mechanics to finish with a tune-up.

Basic Maintenance

You want to keep your bike clean and keep the chain lubricated. To help with the cleaning, keep a collection of old rags handy and purchase a good degreaser (you can find the latter at auto part or bike shops). A degreaser helps with cleaning your chain and anything else that may be greasy.

One way to clean your chain is to wet a rag with a degreaser, lightly grip the chain with the rag, and then turn the pedal backward. Be sure to turn the pedal enough times so the chain makes a full rotation and each link of the chain slides through the rag between your fingers. Use an old toothbrush to get hard-to-reach areas such as chain rings (gears).

When the chain is clean, you'll want to reapply some lubrication. Several types and brands of lube are probably available at the bike store. Don't be overwhelmed by the selection. Some riders like to use a basic oil; others like a wax-based lube. It comes down to price and preference. You might want to try a couple different products to find your favorite, but most likely, you won't notice a difference between any of the standard options.

Blow-Outs

Unfortunately, flat tires happen. The timing can be fickle. Sometimes you'll go for weeks/ months without a flat tire and then bam! You'll get three in a couple days. When it happens and you're riding on clincher tires (standard tire with tube), follow these steps (talk to your local bike shop expert to discuss changing a flat for your race wheel or other specific type of wheel):

1. For a flat on the back tire, shift gears so the back gear is on the smallest ring. This will make it easy to replace the chain when you put the tire back on.

2. Loosen the skewer (the bike's axle) and take the wheel off of the frame. (For the back wheel, this will involve some maneuvering with the chain and gears.)

3. Using the tire valve, release the remaining air from the tire.

4. Insert the flat end of a tire lever (a shoe horn for your tire) between the rim and the tire.

5. Push the other end of the lever down until there's a gap between the rim and the tire, and hook the lever onto a spoke.

6. Place the flat end of the second tire lever into that gap, and start sliding it around the rim.

7. Work the second lever all the way around the full tire until it's back near the first lever and one full side of the tire is off the wheel.

8. Pull the old tube out starting directly opposite the valve. (Put the tube in a back jersey pocket to patch later or discard.)

9. Gently run your fingers along the inside of the tire to locate any potential causes of the flat.

10. Pump a couple strokes of air into the new tube to make the refitting easier (if you have a frame or floor pump). If not, try to blow some air into the tube to get it started.

11. Feed the valve through the hole in the rim.

12. Using your hands, fit the tube around the rim. (Be sure you don't get your hand or fingers pinched between the tire and rim.)

13. Start pushing the tire back on the rim by hand, starting on one side and working your way out from that spot in both directions.

14. When the tire gets taut toward the end, you might need the tire lever to pop it into place. (Be careful not to pinch the tube.)

15. Inflate the tire using your pump or CO_2 cartridge.

16. Remount the wheel.

If you've never changed a flat before, practice doing it at home first before you hit the road.

Coaches' Corner

There are two kinds of bike tube valves: a Presta, or European valve, is long and skinny and is usually used on road bikes; a Shrader, or American valve, looks like a car tire's valve. Some Presta valves are longer than others to accommodate a specific rim. Tire and tube sizes and dimensions vary from bike to bike. Sometimes the numbers appear in millimeters and sometimes in inches. Write down your size somewhere so you don't forget it next time you have to get a tube replacement. Or simply take the old tube to the bike shop when you need a new one.

Get Dialed In

Getting "dialed in" or getting the proper bike fit is crucial. This ensures that you're riding in comfort and with efficiency—both underscored by the reduced chance of injury.

While performing a bike fit, several things can be adjusted to make the bike align to your specific body type. We're going to cover the basics and help you get into the standard, or neutral position, and then you can tweak the position yourself for comfort and aerodynamics.

 Training Tips _____

If you don't feel confident or comfortable with the setup, you might want to consider making an appointment with a certified bike-fitting specialist. A session can take between 1 and 4 hours and might cost mucho dinero. If you decide to go with a professional, keep in mind it will cost a bit now, but you might greatly reduce time, energy, and costs later associated with aches, pains, and injury.

If you'll be using clipless pedals, you first need to get that part of your ride going. As we briefly mentioned in Chapter 3, three main components enable you to use clipless pedals: shoes, pedals, and cleats (in most cases, these are all sold separately). Our first task is to screw the cleats into the correct position on the shoe. The cleat should be directly under the ball of your foot. To be sure it's attached in the right spot, put on your bike shoes. On the inside of the shoe, mark the spot with a pen where you feel the ball of your foot. Line the center of the cleat up with the mark you just made, and screw it into the shoe.

Training Tips _____

If you have trouble picturing 10 or 30 degrees, you can always buy a cheap plastic protractor for a couple bucks (that will bring back some memories of geometry!).

With the cleats set up, we're ready to move onto the saddle height. The goal here is to have your leg bent at 10 to 30 degrees when the pedal is at the lowest possible position. You don't want your legs to ever be fully extended while riding. Your leg should just be short of full extension when in the 6 o'clock position. When you feel like you have the right height, mark where the saddle stem enters the frame with masking tape. Try the bike out for a while at this height. If you feel you're rocking in the saddle when you ride, it may be too high. If you feel pain in your knee due to inadequate leg extension, it may be too low. Tweak the height until you find the sweet spot.

The next piece of the saddle puzzle is to be sure your seat is adjusted forward or backward into a position that maximizes your power. When your front pedal is in the maximum forward position, your knee should be directly above it. To check this, create a simple plumb line. Get a length of string (a bit longer than the length of your leg from your knee to your foot) and attach a metal nut to one end (or anything with some weight such as a pen). While sitting on the bike with your pedals at the 3 and 9 o'clock positions, dangle the plumb line from the side of your knee—use the boney knob, which is the head of the fibula. The nut on the other end of the string should hit the pedal axle. If the nut is in front of the axle, adjust your seat backward a tad. If the nut is behind the axle, move the seat forward a bit. Each time you make an adjustment, recheck using the plumb line test until you're right on.

Your saddle itself should be parallel (or almost parallel) to the ground. After you try it in the parallel position, you might want to make slight adjustments for comfort over time. For example, pointing the nose of the saddle down a fuzz can add comfort for some. However, you don't want to feel like you're slipping forward when you ride.

Your handlebar height should be near level in relation to the saddle. This is considered the neutral position. You can measure this using a yardstick and a carpenter's level. Extend the yardstick out from the top of the saddle and level it up. Then measure the distance between the handlebars and the yardstick. Make slight changes to the height up or down for comfort over time. Keep in mind that every time the handlebars are lowered, the riding position is considered more aggressive. This may be slightly more aerodynamic, but it also puts more strain on your lower back. A setup with the handlebars level or slightly higher than the seat is more comfortable for most riders.

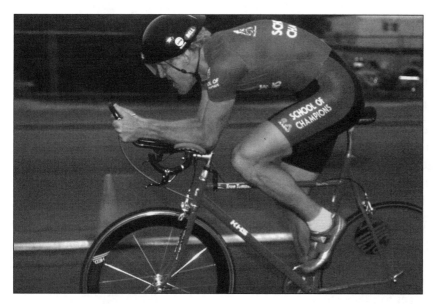

Cycling legend John Howard shows great form in his aggressive bike fit. Note that his handlebars are lower than his seat, his extended leg is still slightly bent, and his upper arms are almost vertical.

(Photo by Lois Schwartz)

Must-Have Preride Checklist

With the bike all set up, you should be close to going out for your first ride. Before you do, though, review this checklist of items we never ride without (don't miss the *'d items!):

- ❏ Saddle bag or other storage pouch
- ❏ Spare tube(s)*
- ❏ Tire levers (two or three)
- ❏ Frame pump or CO_2 cartridges*
- ❏ CO_2 valve adapter (if using cartridges)
- ❏ Multi-purpose compact bike tool (contains Allen wrenches, screwdrivers, etc.)*
- ❏ Cash*

- ❏ Water bottle cages or some kind of hydration system*
- ❏ Energy bars/gels or other nutrition
- ❏ Map of the area
- ❏ Sunglasses*
- ❏ Helmet*
- ❏ Gloves (sometimes)
- ❏ Cycling jersey and shorts
- ❏ Bike shoes and socks

Gravel Ahead

If you're new to having your shoes snapped into the pedals, do not head straight onto the roads, as this could be extremely dangerous. Spend some time riding in a large, traffic-free area such as an off-hours parking lot. Practice clipping in and out of the pedals until it becomes second nature. This will help you avoid anxiety and falls later while you're in the middle of an intersection.

Safety Check

Above all, train safe. Biking involves moving parts, unknown road conditions, and high speeds to contend with. We're not saying something bad will happen; we're just saying that the bike segment can present some precarious situations. Stay vigilant, and you'll be fine.

Keep an eye out for sewer grates—some grates may run parallel to your bike's tire path and your tire could fall into the gaps. If you come across other types of grates, such as a cattle grate, don't panic. These typically run perpendicular to the flow of traffic, and you can safely ride over these types. Anytime you come up to a railroad track, use caution as well. Check for a train and then ride with care over the tracks, making sure to keep your tires perpendicular to the tracks.

Always stay in control while you're riding, and don't let your riding exceed your ability. Don't ride on paths where you need to "thread the needle" (keep your wheels within a very narrow space only a few inches wide). And don't fly down hills at light-speed if you'll have to stop or take a corner when you get to the bottom.

Training Tips _____

To stay in control when you're heading into a sharp turn at high speeds, gradually apply your brakes *prior* to the turn rather than fully squeezing your brakes at the last second. If the grade of the hill is really steep, the majority of the braking should be done using the rear brake. Additionally, when you're heading into a sharp turn, always keep your inside leg up and your outside leg down. This helps you balance and keeps your foot from catching the ground as you lean into the turn.

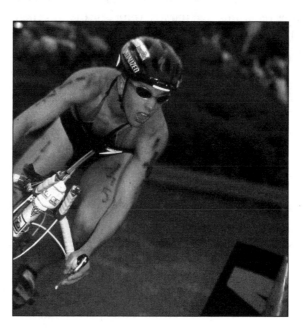

In a sharp turn, this tri-athlete gets out of the aero position, applies slight pressure on the brakes, and keeps his "inside" leg raised.

(Photo by Lois Schwartz)

Rules of the Road

When you ride your bike on a road, you're just like any other vehicle sharing the pavement. You're entitled to the same rights and must abide by the same rules. As a cyclist, you need to be even more aware of traffic and everything around you than other drivers in vehicles.

Communicating your intentions on the road is imperative. Some cyclists follow the traditional hand-turn signals, while others simply point in the direction they are turning. The important thing is that all the other people on the road know what you are going to do. Get in the habit of signaling, even when you think you're alone on the road. It will become second nature after a while, and will help keep you safe in the long run.

Training Tips _____

When cycling on the road, it's safest to ride *with* traffic. You are a vehicle out on the road and need to follow the standard laws. Plus, riding with traffic gives drivers on your side of the road the maximum amount of time to see you before they're upon you. Riding against traffic decreases closure time between you and an oncoming car, giving each of you less time to react to the other.

Use the Buddy System

It's a good idea to ride with a buddy or in small groups. That way, if something does go wrong, you've got backup. You're human, so there might be times when you forget to bring something important along on your ride. If alone, they might be pushing their bike back to civilization (if they can't wrangle a rescue from a friend with a cell phone). A 30-mile walk in bike cleats is not something you want to do. Use the buddy system.

The other benefit of riding with others is that it's great for camaraderie and socializing. You can share tips and stories regarding cycling, triathlon, or life in general. We've done some group rides that are filled with conversation and laughter. One specific character we loved to ride with in southern California is like a nonstop, rolling, comedy routine. He tells so many hilarious stories that before we know it, we're done with the ride and our abs have gotten as much of a workout as our legs from all the laughing.

Gravel Ahead _____

Do not talk on the phone or listen to headphones when you're riding in traffic.

If for some reason you're out riding alone, stick to the areas you know. You might also choose to do a loop that keeps you close to home in lieu of a straight out and back. That way you're not as far away from your base. A cell phone becomes even more important if you're riding alone.

Night Riding and Other Special Situation Equipment

Darkness magnifies all the safety issues riders deal with during the day. It'll be harder to spot obstructions in the road, more difficult for drivers to see you, and harder to navigate. Although we don't recommend going nocturnal, some people do it.

If you absolutely need to ride at night, it's important to light up yourself and your path ahead. Wear reflective tape, lights, and reflectors. Most TRI bikes and road bikes don't come with reflectors out of the box, so be sure to add them if you'll be riding at night. If you're shopping for headlights, remember that the helmet-mounted ones shine light on what you're gazing at. The bike-mounted lights give you additional and steady light and are a must. You can position these depending on how fast you're traveling. Keep a backup battery with you, too.

Clear protective eyewear is essential to keep your eyes safe while riding at night. It protects you from wind and anything airborne such as dirt or bugs that could fly into your eyes. During the day, you might see these things coming at you. At night, with your limited field of vision, you could be surprised by a sudden moth in your face.

Riding in the rain is not recommended either. Rain riding presents many of the same problems night riding presents: limited visibility for the rider, difficulty for drivers to see the rider, the tendency to not use protective eyewear, etc. If you do ride in the rain, be sure to wear a light on your back at a minimum, and wear some sort of protective eyewear.

Rain adds two more negatives to your ride. First, the road will be much slicker, especially when you're making turns. And any of the components on your bike that can rust will be endangered. Of course, if you ride in the rain, you should wipe down your bike as soon as you get back to your base. Just be sure to get into all the cracks and crevasses. Additionally, if you've been in some serious rain, you might want to pull the seat post out and tip the bike upside down. Sometimes water can seep into the bike and rust things out.

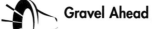

Gravel Ahead

If you're out riding during the rain or anytime it's wet out, be extra careful. The painted street lines can be extremely slippery when wet, especially when you're crossing over one during a turn.

Get to Work: Biking!

To train for the bike portion of triathlon, you'll do several timed bike rides outside. If you have access to some sort of indoor cycle bike, you can do these drills inside.

Single Leg Drills (SLDs)

SLDs are great for developing and improving your "full circle" mentality. On your indoor cycle, sit on the bike and clip one cleat into the pedal. Leave the other cleat out of the pedal and resting on a box or a table out of the way of all moving parts, or hook your toes back on the trainer (but safely away from the spokes and chain). Make it as comfortable as possible. Remember to keep the rest of your body in normal riding line. You don't want the one leg off the bike to throw you out of balance.

Start pedaling in a very easy gear using the one leg. This is the time to really hone in on the technical aspect of your riding. Focus on the full circle, and make things as smooth as possible while keeping the RPM above 80. You can shift as needed.

Training Tips

Drills on a bike trainer are a great way to focus on specific muscle groups and technique in a controlled environment. You can do these workouts in front of a TV, but be sure to keep your intensity where it should be.

Spin with the one leg for a specified time; then clip in the second leg and unclip the first for the same time. Repeat the interval for the specified number of repetitions.

Large Gear Drills (LGDs)

LGDs are performed using both legs in a large gear and at a lower RPM. These intervals are great for increasing muscular strength and endurance. The idea is analogous to weight lifting: the drill is more focused on muscular fitness than cardiovascular endurance. Stay seated, keep it smooth, and focus on the circular motion of each pedal stroke.

Here's an example of this drill: spin in a larger gear for 2 minutes (less than 80 RPM). Recover for a minute in an easy gear (less than 100 RPM) and then repeat the intervals 3 to 5 times.

Small Gear Drills (SGDs)

SGDs are also performed using both legs and really get your legs spinning fast. These speed intervals help develop your neuromuscular system by teaching it to fire efficiently at higher rates. Focus on applying consistent force all the way around the pedal stroke. You want to spin very fast, but if your form starts to suffer, get into a slightly harder gear and back down the RPMs a tad.

> **Coaches' Corner**
>
> While doing these drills, it's very important to maintain good form. If you begin to bounce in the saddle, slow it down.

A sample drill would be to spin at a high RPM (greater than 100) in an easy gear for an interval (60 seconds). Recover for a shorter interval (30 seconds), and repeat 4 or 5 intervals.

Road Training Considerations

The rest of your bike training, weather permitting, will be done out on the road. Here's a quick list of some additional heads-up tips to keep in mind while you're out there:

◆ If you're approaching a bump in the road, lift yourself up off your saddle so you can absorb the impact with your arms and legs (not your butt).

◆ Keep your fingers loose. This helps reduce wasted energy in your hands.

◆ If your feet start to tingle, wiggle your toes and be sure your shoes aren't too tight. You might be experiencing poor circulation.

◆ When you first start cycling, you might notice your butt getting sore from the saddle. Don't panic; it will get better over time, as that area gets "conditioned." Applying a pain-relieving cream might help. We find those containing arnica particularly effective.

Vary It Up

The duration, intensity, and terrain of your rides will vary depending on your goals and your environment. However, generally speaking, you should plan to incorporate variety in your training. Most triathletes we know get their cycling conditioning in many ways such as slow-long-flat rides, steady-moderate pace rolling rides, interval type hill/descend rides, mixed terrain and pace rides, indoor cycling classes, turbo-trainer bike rides, and off-road mountain bike rides. You can try countless combinations, and we give suggestions in your training schedules (see Chapters 13 and 14).

Every once in a while, we like to make an adventure of it. We pack up our bikes and drive an hour or so to areas that are beautiful, have low traffic, and are challenging. We pack a lunch and bring along a camera. We don't get to do this every day, but doing something like this occasionally can be very refreshing. The objective is to keep things interesting, safe, and fun. Enjoy the journey!

The Least You Need to Know

- Pedal in a full-circle motion and in the right cadence (80 to 100 RPMs) to improve efficiency.
- Ride with the right equipment at all times: helmet, sunglasses, sun block, etc.
- A good bike fit enhances your form and helps reduce your chance of injury.
- Always ride with a buddy for safety and support.
- Vary your training to keep things from getting stale and also promote growth.

Chapter 7

Running Down Your Dream

In This Chapter

♦ Understanding the benefits of taking to the track (or the treadmill)

♦ Improving on your form

♦ Increasing your speed

The versatility of running makes it one of the greatest sports. All you need are shoes, and off you go. Not only does running help make you fit, but it's also one of the best ways to explore your surroundings. You might be surprised at what you discover both in your neck of the woods as well as while visiting other towns and cities in your travels. And by the way, the "runner's high" is not a myth.

The Benefits of Running

Running is a superb cardiovascular exercise. Few other fitness activities can elevate your heart rate so effectively as running. There's no faking it with running. You're propelling your full body weight forward the entire time you're working out. That helps you gain cardiovascular fitness. That helps you gain strength.

Most people who don't exercise regularly find running almost offensive. If you ask them to go for a run, their faces screw up like they just tasted some super-sour pickle. What's the root cause of this tremendous dislike? We believe it starts as kids with physical education class and other sports. In both gym class and practices for sports like soccer, football, baseball, etc., young people are forced to practice running as a part of the workout for some other sport ("Go run 10 laps and then we'll work on hitting"). It's even sometimes used as punishment ("Run 15 sprints after practice"). Although this makes perfect sense from a teacher's or coach's perspective, something negative happens in the young mind. Psychologists call this "association."

Kids want to go play soccer or football or softball ... but someone first makes them go through this running routine their body dislikes. They eventually grow up, perhaps without specific memories of running but knowing that timed running was the painful part of something they otherwise enjoyed doing.

Coaches' Corner

How do you feel about running? Really think about it for a minute. At the thought of running, do you have a happy feeling filled with sunshine and beautiful trails? Or do you picture a field you have to run around *X* number of times in the rain before you can start practice? If you're in the first group, you are ready to go! If you're in the second group, let's get you over those negative feelings right quick: you are now going to be running with serious purpose.

We'll be using running to train specifically to become a better runner, ergo a better triathlete. Think about that: we're not going to go out and run because Coach said we had to if we want to make next year's soccer team. We're doing it so that when we are on our last leg of our triathlon, we're going to be prepared. We're going to be ready to keep striding along because we have practiced and our body is ready to run. Try to free your mind and allow yourself to reevaluate running for what it is: an extremely beneficial cardio workout that's going to play a crucial role in your triathlon training. Start out slow and build your way up. Think baby steps. You can do this.

Do It Anywhere

Running is the perfect fitness exercise because location is not a limiting factor. People can run anywhere in the world. Before you start to object, saying your neighborhood has too many hills, is too cold, or is otherwise impossible to run in, consider this: there is a marathon in Antarctica! Most likely, the conditions outside your house or apartment are not quite as severe as near the South Pole! If it's hot, bring some water with you; if it's cold, dress in layers; if there are a lot of hills, go slower and take smaller steps than you would on flat terrain.

Not only does running enable you to get a good workout; it also enables you to explore your surroundings. You'll see things you'd otherwise miss if you were driving in a car or working in an office. Enjoy it. Take in the sights, no matter if they're traditionally picturesque or not. If you're in a new area, be sure to pay careful attention to where you're going—or leave a trail of breadcrumbs, whatever's easier.

Training Tips

Even if you love nature, it's okay to train indoors sometimes. When the temperature reaches extremes, people who exercise in the elements might put themselves in greater danger than the average person. In extreme heat, people may become dehydrated or possibly experience heat cramps, heat exhaustion, or even heat stroke. In extreme cold, frostbite or hypothermia can become risks. When the temperature is really *too* hot or *too* cold, find an indoor alternative for your workout.

No Baggage Required

Racquetball requires a racket, a ball, and a court. Soccer requires a ball and some sort of goals. Biking requires all your cycling equipment. With running, you can elevate your heart rate and fitness level using nothing more than your shoes and your determination. At home, running is nice to do because it doesn't take any preparation time to get ready, and you don't need to drive anywhere. If you're traveling, you only need to bring along your shoes and some workout clothes, and you're ready to run no matter where you end up.

Technically Speaking

Running is really the same as walking, except a bit faster. And it makes it a little harder to breathe. And it might make you sweat as well. And by definition, during your run, at times, you will have neither foot touching the ground (unlike walking, in which you always have at least one foot on the ground). To run, you don't need to learn to use any special equipment. Generally speaking, if you can walk, you can run; the time and distance will come.

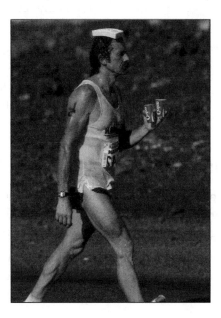

It is absolutely, positively okay to walk.

(Photo by Lois Schwartz)

If running seems a little overwhelming at first, it's okay to walk. In the beginning of your program, you might walk some or most of the minutes in your "run" workout. That's fine. Pausing to walk during a running workout isn't cheating. Almost all runners walk from time to time; it's a great way to break up the work into smaller pieces. In fact, walking can and should be used as part of the warm-up, cool-down, and in between.

There's no magic formula we can tell you to make running an effortless, work-free, fun time. However, we can give you insight that will enable you to make your running more efficient. Running can be a time to think. Let your mind wander—it'll help you pass the miles more easily. However, stay mindful of technique.

One Foot in Front of the Other ... Almost

When running, you want to keep your feet landing slightly in front of you and relatively close to your body's centerline. You don't want to have your feet landing far from that centerline—you'd look like a jogging cowboy who just got off a full day on a horse. You also want to avoid having your feet cross over that centerline (i.e., your right foot land on the left side of that centerline). The latter is virtually impossible, but if this applies to you, you'll want to adjust your form.

Gravel Ahead

Most people experience some soreness when they first start running. That soreness should go away as your muscles become accustomed to the program. If you have some nagging pains that don't feel like regular soreness, get checked out immediately. The fix might be as simple as putting orthotics in your shoes or working on some exercises to strengthen specific muscles.

Keeping your feet landing on or near the centerline helps you in two ways: it creates less stress on your knees, hips, and ankles, and it keeps you from wasting energy on side-to-side movement. If you're not sure how your form stacks up, ask a friend to watch you run or set up a video camera to record your stride while on a treadmill or out on a sidewalk. You'll quickly see if you're landing near the centerline.

Another simple way to analyze your form is to take a look at the bottom of your feet after a few runs or at the bottom of an old pair of running shoes. If you're developing blisters in certain areas or your shoes are worn unevenly, your form probably has a small issue that can be corrected with orthotics.

Perfectly Proper Posture

"Don't slouch!" Your parents might have told you that as a kid. We're telling you again. Good posture while running helps your diaphragm expand fully and deliver the maximum amount of oxygen to your lungs. Running (and more specifically, triathlon) is all about efficiency.

Ideally, you should lean slightly forward at the hips. If you feel like your legs are leading out in front of you, you're not leaning forward far enough. If you feel like you need to keep moving forward just to keep your balance, you're probably leaning too far forward. Find the lean that's just right.

Don't Bounce

You've seen this type of runner before: the bouncer. This runner bounds along with his or her body going up and down as they travel down the street. They look like they might be going up in the air the same distance they're moving forward.

This is not efficient. This is the epitome of *in*efficiency. You don't have to be a physics major to realize that, when running, it's better to expend your energy to create forward motion rather than vertical motion.

Run Relaxed

The majority of your energy should be dedicated toward propelling yourself forward. Any muscles not being used should be as relaxed as possible. Don't flex your arm muscles. Simply have a comfortable bend in the elbow (around 90 degrees), and keep that same bend as your arms move back and forth. And your arms should go straight forward and backward while they're pumping, not *across* your body. Your hands should be relatively loose, as if you're gently holding a potato chip in each one.

> **Training Tips**
>
> To get the correct bend in your arms while running, try to have your fingers brush by the elastic waistband on your shorts with each pump.

One place many runners forget to relax is their face. If you're running while wincing in pain, frowning, or clinching your teeth, you're wasting energy. One of Steve's tricks when he thinks his face might be tense is to smile. Nice and easy, right? Smiling helps loosen the cheek and mouth muscles and initiates his facial relaxation. Try it next time you're out for a run. This technique can help start a chain reaction of relaxation that flows down your body.

Just Breathe

You've been breathing all your life, so why did we write a whole section on doing it? Because when people exercise, they seem to forget how to breathe. They tend to either hold their breath or take abbreviated breaths. If you're just starting out or if you feel like you're always out of breath when you exercise, pay close attention to this section.

Biology tells us that our cells need oxygen to operate properly. Our cells need to receive that oxygen from our blood, which receives O_2 from our lungs. The more oxygen we can get into our lungs, the better off we'll be. Holding your breath or taking short breaths limits the amount of O_2 available for the blood stream. If you've ever been in a weight room, you might have seen someone lifting weights and holding his breath as he pushed. His face probably turned red, veins popped out of his forehead, and when he was done, he was probably breathing hard. This is not safe in any sport.

During most nonspeed workouts, your breathing should be relaxed. It'll be more labored when you're running than when you're lying in bed, obviously, but you shouldn't be gasping. You should be able to carry on a conversation with someone. You don't *need* to talk, but you should have enough oxygen if you wanted to.

> ### Coaches' Corner
>
> Colin and one of his triathlon mentors, Donna, came up with a nickname for this measure of breathing: the Cubs game talk test. If Colin is running at a good pace and his breathing is smooth and deep enough, he should be able to talk about how his favorite baseball team is doing. Use this idea in your own runs. Even if you're running alone, you can test your exertion levels by monologuing about anything that interests you. Or speak the lyrics of a song or recite some poetry you were forced to memorize in school. Don't worry about any strange looks you might receive; people should be used to this sort of thing in the age of cell-phone earpieces.

The point is this: if you can't catch your breath while you're talking during a normal run, you're pushing too hard.

Cadence Check

Higher cadence means higher efficiency. Nobody runs a race of any distance with long jump strides; likewise, no one runs with baby steps. The perfect cadence is somewhere in between. If your cadence is more along the lines of the quicker, shorter strides, your muscles delay fatigue and your breathing flows more smoothly.

A faster cadence means your feet are touching the ground more times per minute, too. The time spent in the air isn't making you go faster at all. With each push off from the ground, you're propelling yourself forward. Keep your leg turnover high, and you'll stay efficient.

Roll On

Your foot might hit the ground in one of three ways. Most people land on their heel, roll their foot toward the front, and then push off with their toes. Others strike with their midfoot, roll forward a bit, and push off on their toes. Most elite athletes land on their forefoot and then push off almost immediately. When you're just starting out, you shouldn't worry too much about what kind of foot strike you have. Just go with the flow and try to concentrate on the other checkpoints of your form. However, the more forward you can land on your foot, the less forward momentum you'll lose each step.

Heel striking is equivalent to putting on the brakes a little bit with each step. Think about a sprinter or go out and do a little sprint yourself: when sprinting very fast, you're up on your toes, spending very little time per foot on the ground and keeping a high turnover. When you get to the end of the sprint and want to slow down, you lengthen your stride and reach with your heel for several steps until you stop. You don't keep up on your toes and try to slow down with that form.

If you are a bona fide heel striker and want to transition to a forefoot striker, take your time. There's a big difference between the two running styles, and making the transition will probably stress your feet and lower legs. If you go this route, try to run on soft surfaces and allow for ample recovery between runs. Additionally, work on increasing your cadence, as your stride will naturally shorten and probably bring your strike closer to the front of your foot.

Let's regroup with a list of things to remember regarding your running. Try to remember and run through this list several times during your next run:

- Stand tall.
- Don't bounce.
- Run relaxed.
- Just breathe.
- Keep a quicker cadence.
- Land on your forefoot.

The Mental Game

In running, especially for people who are not elite athletes, the mental aspect is huge. We can't stress enough the importance of having a positive mental attitude as you're running. Where your mind leads, your body truly will follow. Don't say to yourself, *I'm going to try to run four miles today.* Instead, proclaim, *I am going to run four miles today.* Believe in yourself. Believe you can do this. Remove all doubt, and if some tries to surface, just ask yourself, *Why* can't *I do this?* You'll find there's no reason.

> **Training Tips**
>
> Running has been found to boost levels of a natural anti-depressant called phynylacetic acid. Eat your heart out, Prozac; we're going for a run.

Every once in a while, Colin catches himself in a poor mental place regarding running. Usually it occurs when the weather is less than ideal outside and he has elected to use a treadmill. If he starts off thinking, *I'll try to run for forty minutes,* he is constantly checking the time and thinking about how much longer he *has* to run. However, when he goes in with a positive attitude and thinks, *I'm going to run forty minutes,* the time goes by smoothly. Attitude is everything.

Where Should I Run?

Anywhere! The keys to deciding where to run are (1) is it safe? and (2) can I find my way around? You don't need to know exact distances; your watch will guide you.

Keep a couple things in mind when deciding where to run:

- Less traffic = fewer interruptions of your run.
- Well lit = less chance of a twisted ankle.

The first one is a no-brainer. Your parents probably told you to "Watch out for cars!" constantly as you were growing up. You learned that the fewer cars around, the safer you would be (or at least the less you'd be yelled at). The same principle applies here. Running in downtown Chicago or New York might seem like a nice idea, but then you realize that the city streets force you to stop every few hundred feet because of cross traffic. Not to mention taxis and other hurried drivers aren't necessarily looking for runners when they're rushing to make a quick turn. When possible, choose a spot with the least amount of traffic.

Lighting is worth mentioning, although most people usually don't choose to go out and run in the dark. What's far more likely is that a runner will go out for a workout without figuring out how many daylight hours are left until sunset. Only after it's too late will he or she realize that the sun is going to beat them home. Running in the dark is dangerous because you can hurt yourself by twisting an ankle or running into something you couldn't see. You're also more at risk for being unseen by a motorist. Your smartest bet is, of course, to run when there's ample light you know will last your entire run. If you think there's a chance darkness could set in before your run is finished, run with flashing red running lights attached to your front and back. Although this won't help illuminate your way, it will make you more visible to others.

> ### Training Tips
>
> When you are or might soon be running in an environment that's not well lit and shared by other people or motorists, light yourself up! You can find flashing red LED running lights at almost any sporting goods store. They're slightly larger than a silver dollar, very light, cost only a few dollars, and can clip onto almost anything. Use them for any early morning workouts when the sun is still rising and any early evening workouts when you're trying to beat the sunset.

If you must run in the dark because of job constraints or other reasons, you need to be able to clearly see your path. Some companies have started to develop flashlights specifically for runners that illuminate both the path in front you as well as the ground at your feet. These devices cannot illuminate the path as well as daylight, but they're much better than running in the dark.

Get Out and Enjoy Nature (If You Can)

Working out in the great outdoors can be wonderful. Most people are cooped up in an office or other place of business all day during the workweek. Running gives us all an excuse to get outside, breathe fresh air, and soak in the sunshine.

There's never a shortage of places you can go run. Roads, sidewalks, and forest preserves all over the country await you. Your path ahead may be concrete, asphalt, crushed limestone, dirt, grass, or any other surface. The softer the surface, the less impact on your body, specifically your feet, knees, and back. The harder the surface, the faster you'll go. We definitely recommend trading in some speed for less impact on your joints when you can.

Trail running is highly recommended because of its lower impact than harder surfaces and, believe it or not, because of its uneven footing. It sounds crazy, but studies have found that because trails aren't completely level, your legs actually get a benefit from running on these terrains. The little uneven surfaces of the trail help build up the small stabilizer muscles in your feet and ankles.

If you do choose to hit some trails, be sure to take into consideration some extra precautions:

- As always, run with someone else whenever possible.

- Bring everything you might need, as there may be no water or bathroom breaks on the trail.

- Be sure your shoes have some support.

- Map out your route beforehand if it's a documented trail system, and keep track of where you're going.

- Check ahead of time for any sort of warnings in the area (flash floods, wild animals, etc.).

> **Training Tips**
>
> When approaching a hill, keep your head up and your eyes focused on the crest of it. This helps open your airways, which makes it easier to breathe and to reach the top.

> **Coaches' Corner**
>
> As a kid, you probably never needed an excuse to run. Today, however, you might. Don't let a case of seasonal affective disorder get you. Head out for a run!

Even if you can't find trails in your area, you can emulate trails by running on grass or dirt that runs parallel to a sidewalk or road. You might not want to run on the grass of a neighbor who meticulously manicures the lawn twice a day, but we're sure you can find some spots that allow you to get some low-impact workouts.

Track It Down

If you have access to—and feel more comfortable running on—an outdoor track, go for it! Tracks usually are made of materials softer than concrete, and that helps keep the impact on your body low. Some people like tracks because they can be sure of the exact distance they run during a workout. (Neither of us keep track of how many laps we've done; we usually go by time/duration.)

The downfall of tracks is the constant turning. On a quarter-mile track, a 3-mile run includes 1.5 miles of soft turns. Because our legs are designed to run in a straight line, turning this much in one direction can be harmful. One way to minimize the negative impact of this turning (or at least share the impact between both sides of the legs) is to reverse positions fairly often. One lap in each direction is ideal for the legs, but breaks up your rhythm very frequently. Two and two, or four and four, etc., would work, too.

> **Gravel Ahead**
>
> Recently, cold and wet weather struck when Steve had a run workout scheduled. He decided to take it to his local fitness center and train using its small track. After only 20 minutes, his knees and Achilles' tendons were nagging.

If you can, stay away from extremely short tracks such as indoor tracks. These tracks force runners to go around 10 or more times just to run a single mile, and the angles can put too much stress on joints, muscles, tendons, and ligaments. (Remember "runner's knee" from Chapter 4.) Even if you try to reverse your direction every so often to minimize the impact, doing so on such a short track will surely make your head spin! Short tracks should be your very last option for workouts, and if used, should be done so very sparingly.

Treadmills

Treadmills are nice alternatives for people who want to avoid inclement weather or can't normally run during daylight hours. They're also the perfect fit for people with bad knees or those who are carrying around a few extra pounds. A treadmill's running surface is softer than any type of natural ground and absorbs much of the impact from running.

Treadmills can teach you pacing consistency. If you set the machine to give you a 30-minute workout at 10 minutes per mile, barring any manual adjustment on your part, you'll run exactly 10-minute miles. This is also a downside to treadmills: they may condition you to expect consistency. The probability that your triathlon will involve a perfectly flat, entirely straight, weatherless run is next to nothing. Even indoor triathlons involve turns around the track. If you do prefer running on treadmills to running outdoors, still be sure you incorporate several outdoor runs into your schedule before the big day. You don't want get into the run portion of a triathlon and be surprised that wind and hills actually do make a difference in your running! At a minimum, you should run with a 1 percent incline, as discussed in Chapter 3.

Although treadmills have a fairly basic concept, they can vary greatly from brand to brand. Some have variable inclines and several "programs" you can utilize to emulate a hill workout or a speed workout. The key factor is that you learn how to use the machine before you're in the middle of a workout. Locate the emergency stop button before turning anything on. Hopefully, you'll never need it, but better safe than sorry.

Gravel Ahead _____

Some people become lulled by treadmills. They always run at a constant pace with no incline and the treadmill just "pulling" them along. In the real world, they find their pace much slower. Don't let this happen to you! Always run with at least some incline, and be sure to vary your speed every once in a while. If your machine doesn't allow you to mechanically vary the incline, we're confident you can figure out a safe way to make it happen manually.

Also be sure you understand how to increase and decrease the speed and incline of the treadmill before starting a workout. If you do a hill workout, be aware that although the incline of the treadmill base increases, the speed most likely stays the same. If you're running outside and you hit a hill, your speed will naturally decrease. A treadmill doesn't account for this, so be prepared to manually slow your speed as the incline increases.

Safety Check

Running on a treadmill presents a few mechanical hazards, but running outdoors has some dangers as well. The best advice we can give you is to use common sense. Be safe and have a plan:

◆ Take pepper spray if you're running alone.

◆ Bring a cell phone and some emergency cash.

◆ Know (at least generally) where you're headed.

◆ Know how to get back to where you started.

◆ Bring water and food if the duration you're going necessitates it.

◆ If you have to run on a street, run *against* traffic. That way, you can keep your eye on the vehicles coming at you instead of turning your back on them.

Remember in Chapter 6 when we talked about riding with the traffic? Running is the opposite. Running toward traffic doesn't significantly decrease closure time between you and any cars, but it does give you great visibility as to what is coming your way. If you're out on the road and not on a trail, head toward the flow of traffic. Keep off the road if at all possible. Stay as far left as possible; in a shoulder or on the side walk.

The words pepper spray bring up visuals of dark parking lots or late-night city streets. That's not the only place where the stuff can come in handy, though. We're not trying to cause unnecessary panic here; we're just trying to be sure you're as safe as possible. Pepper spray is easy to carry and can save your life if used correctly. You'll be able to find it in most specialty stores. And we're not talking only to women here. Men who are running alone are usually less likely targets than women, but that doesn't guarantee a man's safety.

Whenever possible, train with a buddy. It'll add camaraderie, encouragement, and safety to your workout. The buddy system is always encouraged in all forms of exercise, from swimming to weight lifting, and running is no different. However, we know that it's not always possible to find a running partner who shares your exact same fitness schedule or level. Don't sweat it. Try to work out with a buddy whenever you can, but if that's not possible, or you just feel like working out on your own at certain points, go for it. Just use your head. Have your phone and pepper spray handy, and be sure someone knows where you're headed and when you'll be back.

Training Tips

You could probably chase away a little yappy dog on your own, but with a big dog, you'll be happy to have pepper spray. Be prepared.

Get to Work: Running!

People have been running for thousands of years. Luckily for all of us, we can stand on the shoulders of giants to maximize our performance. We'll look at several types of runs to incorporate into our workouts: long runs, transition runs, and speed workouts.

This is not an all-inclusive list of the types of running workouts you could do, but these are the major types we're going to cover. They'll be more than enough to get you ready for your triathlon.

Going Long

Colin's girlfriend is a marathon runner who used to despise running. She felt that a long run was anything longer than a 100-meter dash. After being inspired by watching the Ironman in Hawaii, she decided to take up running. After starting off very slowly, she currently uses phrases like "… only 14 miles" when referring to her training schedule. Colin smiles to remember the old Bonnie.

Long runs are any distance or time that makes you think, *Wow! I'm going to run for* X *minutes?!* Everything is relative: if you've never run before and thought you never would, a long run might be 20 minutes. If you're already logging 45 minutes every morning on the treadmill before work, a 90-minute run might be your definition of *long*. We'll call it a long run when its duration is longer than the other runs during that week. Typically, there's only one of these workouts in your schedule per week.

Transition Runs

Transition runs (T-runs) are those you run within a few minutes after completing a bike workout. Don't get nervous about this and think it's beyond you. All you're doing is helping condition your body to do what it'll need to do in the race: transition from cycling to running. Your leg muscles need to get used to going from the circular pedal stroke to a running rhythm/movement.

Preparing for a T-run helps you practice what to bring on the day of the race. There's no better way to find out that you forgot to include something vital than to do it during a training workout. Before leaving for your ride, lay out all the equipment and food you'll want to take on your T-run. These things should really be no different from what you bring on a normal run. After your workout, make notes about how the transition went: what you did well and what you need to improve on. Maybe you had all the equipment you needed but you completely forgot to put out extra water to rehydrate while you were changing shoes. Make a note, and do it better the next time.

> **Coaches' Corner**
>
> T-runs will seem awkward at first. Give it time, and they'll begin to feel normal. You'll do so many of these during training that it will be almost like second nature during a race.

I Feel the Need, the Need for Speed!

You shouldn't do speed workouts until you've established a strong base, like we talked about in Chapter 4. Including speed workouts into a training program too early—like trying any other fitness-related activities too early—can overstress your body and/or cause injury. Our programs start to build speed work in after about a month of training. This way, our bodies have the chance to get used to triathlon before pushing them to the next level. Each speed workout is sandwiched between a warm-up to get the blood flowing before the session and a cool-down afterward.

The best-named speed workout is the *fartlek*. Fartlek is Swedish for "speed play." A fartlek workout involves a warm-up and then a series of periods where you pick up speed. After each pick-up, you go back to the regular speed; after you've done your designated number of pick-ups, you can finish your run.

The pick-up during a fartlek is *not* a sprint. You don't want to push your body to the breaking point. You're simply picking up the pace for a bit and then going back to your normal speed. The period used can be marked by feel, distance, or time. Steve prefers to do his fartleks by feel, speeding up when he feels ready and then backing off to a normal speed when his body tells him to. Colin prefers to use some sort of markers like city blocks in his neighborhood or street signs as indicators of when to pick it up and slow down. The beauty of this type of run is that you can make it into whatever you want!

Coaches' Corner

You might be reading this book because you want to get to the finish line of your very first TRI. You want to avoid the hype, avoid any hassle along the way, and just finish a race in whatever time it takes. So right now you might be thinking *I don't feel the need for speed at all!* That's understandable. Many beginners want to leave speed work out of their program all together. We know you're probably not planning on winning your race, but speed work helps you live up to your fullest potential and also breaks up the monotony of going out and running *X* minutes. We highly recommend you try a few. You might just enjoy yourself.

Tempo runs consist of a warm-up, an up-pace run, and a cool-down. The up-pace portion of this workout is, again, not a sprint, but simply a bit of a pick-up from your normal pace. With this speed workout, however, you should calculate the full distance you'll run as precisely as possible, as well as at least four intermediate distances. This enables you to confirm that your pace is consistent throughout the run (i.e., for a mile pick-up at a 10-minute-mile pace, each quarter mile should be 2 minutes, 30 seconds). You can measure exact distances by using your bike or car's odometer or by running on a track. You could also use a heart-rate monitor with a built-in speed-tracking feature.

The first time you do this sort of workout, you might want to try just a half-mile tempo run. Start out slow and be sure you stay consistent; consistency trumps speed. Your warm-up and cool-down will be around 10 to 15 minutes each and should increase as the tempo run distance increases. A good rule of thumb is to keep the tempo run distance about the same distance as your warm-up distance.

Intervals might leave a bad taste in your mouth if you ever had a track coach who pushed you to the limit. This workout involves a warm-up and then several "intervals" of fast-paced running over a specific distance/time, with plenty of rest in between. During the rest, an extremely slow jog is recommended, although walking is permitted at the start of the rest period. The interval distances/times can vary depending on the training plan you're going for.

def•i•ni•tion

Fartleks (Swedish for "speed play") involve a warm-up and then a series of shorter, up-paced periods, defined by distance between landmarks (city blocks), time, or general feel. This is not a very regimented workout. **Tempo runs** feature a warm-up and then the tempo is increased to a faster-than-normal pace and sustained for the designated period of time. Usually done on a track, **interval** workouts involve several periods of high intensity with a designated period of recovery. The periods are usually marked by distance on a track but can be marked by time as well.

Initially, most workouts are based on running (or running/walking) for a specific amount of time. Distance is not nearly as important as the amount of time you put in. After you establish a base and are ready for some speed work, you'll start to incorporate fartleks, tempo runs, and intervals. A sample interval workout might include a 10- to 15-minute warm-up and then 4 faster 400-meter (or the equivalent amount of time it takes you to run a faster than normal 400) intervals, each with about a minute rest in between. Follow the speed workout with a cool-down.

Just for the Drill of It

The last thing we're going to mention to help improve your speed are drills and accelerations. These two techniques are not workouts in and of themselves; they're more like the icing on the cake at the end of a run session. Both drills and accelerations help increase your foot turnover and, therefore, your speed. These are not difficult to do, but the payoff can be tremendous. Although Colin never liked the distance training he did in high school, he loved doing stride outs and drills because they were short, fun, and, at times, goofy.

All you need to do drills and accelerations is a straight, flat area where you can run unimpeded for about 100 yards (give or take a few). Our favorite surfaces are dirt trails or tracks, but flat grassy areas or bump-free sidewalks can work, too. Just be sure to examine the area first so you aren't surprised by any uneven ground. You can choose to do each of your drills for a number of repetitions (20 each leg) or for a specific distance (from the edge of the sidewalk to that tree over there).

We could overwhelm you with several drills, but we'll just look at four:

- Butt kicks

- High knees

- Side-stepping cross-overs

- Skipping

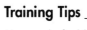

Training Tips _____

You might feel like you look funny while doing drills, but don't worry about what other people think. The benefits are worth any inquisitive looks you might receive from the neighbors.

These, with accelerations, will definitely improve your speed.

Butt kicks—the name just implies fun, doesn't it? In this simple drill, you work on the part of your stride that's behind the midpoint of your body. You should already be warmed up from your main running workout. From your "starting line," you can take a couple steps to get moving. Then, while continuing to run, try to kick up one of your heels and hit your butt. Repeat with the other foot. When this serious butt kicking is going on, your feet will be moving quickly off the ground but you won't be moving forward that quickly. That's fine. Don't worry if your heel isn't actually touching your butt in the kick. The important thing to improve your speed is to get the essence of the motion right.

High knees keep your feet moving at the same speed as butt kicks, but your focus shifts to keeping your legs in front of you (instead of behind you). Simply take a couple steps and then start lifting those knees! You might feel like a soldier marching in double time, and you'll probably need to lean back a bit to balance yourself. Don't try to lift your knees so high that you risk pulling something. Keep yourself in control the entire time.

Side-stepping cross-overs, or "karaoke" as Colin's track coach used to call them, are a great way to get some of your leg stabilization muscles firing. The movement is similar to the sideways movements in some line dances (it's electric! boogie woogie woogie!) except your foot speed is much faster. Here are the steps:

1. Hold your arms out to your sides for stabilization.

2. Take a sidestep to the right with your right foot.

3. Bring your left foot over the right and plant it.

4. Take another sidestep to the right with your right foot.

5. Bring your left foot behind the right and land.

Gravel Ahead _____

Side-stepping cross-overs require a little coordination, so take your time getting used to the mechanics of this drill. Don't rush it and trip over your own feet!

Repeat steps 2 though 5 until you cover your goal distance or number of steps. Then, head back to the left side doing the opposite thing.

Skipping is another fun drill. This time you're working on the front part of your stride. Even if you don't know how to skip in the traditional sense, the exaggerated movement we show you will teach you in no time. Again, you can begin from your "starting line" with a few steps of jogging. Then, whenever you decide, instead of putting your foot down immediately after bringing it forward in a stride, raise one of your knees as high as you can. At the same time, raise your opposite arm (same symmetry as when you're running normally). The momentum of your raising knee and your raising arm causes you to rise a bit off the ground with your back leg. Then, when your first leg comes down, repeat the same motion with the opposite leg. You're skipping just like a kid.

Accelerations are exactly what they sound like. Instead of running at a constant speed, you accelerate for a given distance (100 meters or less; about the distance of a football/soccer field). Don't worry if you think this sounds tough; we promise it isn't that bad. With this drill, you start off with a slower pace and then speed up a bit. Then after a few more steps, accelerate a bit more.

At no time should you be in an all-out sprint, but by the end, you should be running much faster than normal. When you hit the "finish line," slow down until you're either jogging or walking. Catch your breath for a bit at the finish line and then turn around and do another acceleration in the opposite direction. You could also jog or walk to the "starting line" as your breather and do your next acceleration in the same direction. Start off doing four of these after a workout and quickly build up to six.

With long, low-intensity runs, mixed in with speed workouts and drills, you'll see your running improving in no time at all.

The Least You Need to Know

◆ You can run almost anywhere with very little "equipment."

◆ A positive mental attitude goes a long way in your running program—consistency and performance.

◆ You can always tweak your form for maximum efficiency.

◆ Fartleks, tempo runs, and intervals will be difficult at first but will make you a stronger runner.

◆ Accelerations and drills help improve your speed.

Chapter 8

Shifting Gears: Transitions

In This Chapter

- ◆ Understanding why smooth transitions are so important
- ◆ Transition checklists
- ◆ Successful transitions: it's all about attitude

Your race is going to consist of three disciplines (swim, bike, run), held together with a few transition minutes to change equipment, muscle groups, and mind-set. Changing equipment during all the excitement can be a little rough. Using different muscle groups and adopting a new perspective while starting the bike or run can be even more challenging.

But don't worry. You'll be prepared because we're going to help you practice transitions in your regular workouts. When race day comes, you'll be ready.

Transitions: The Glue That Holds the Sport Together

Some TRI newbies go to their first race without ever considering how to get from one sport to the next. They might have practiced all three sports enough to succeed in them individually, but the transition might cause some confusion.

The concept of a transition is really not that difficult. All you need to do is …

1. Find your gear within the transition area.
2. Drop off the equipment you no longer need.
3. Pick up the equipment you need for the next segment.

The key is to bring everything you need and everything you think you *might* need. It's better to be overprepared than underprepared. If you decide in the middle of the race that you don't need something, you can always leave it behind.

> ### Coaches' Corner
>
> In a race, the transitions are numbered based on their sequence. Your first transition, or T1, is between the swim and the bike. Your second transition, or T2, ties together the bike and the run.

Without a little guidance and forward thinking, your first few transitions might be a little hard to get through. Don't overcomplicate things. All you have to do is be sure you lay out all the gear you'll need for the *next* sport in a specific spot. When you come in from the *previous* event and complete your transition, the spot for your *next* sport should be void of gear.

T1: Swim to Bike

When finishing a swim workout, how do you usually feel? We bet you're wet, thirsty, and maybe hungry. Maybe you also have to go to the bathroom. Those are the four main things to mark off the list during T1.

During a race, most people choose to air dry to avoid spending time toweling off. During a swim-to-bike transition workout, you might decide you want to dry yourself a bit before mounting up. If so, have a towel handy in your transition area.

Most people find that it's difficult to eat anything right after the swim. If you're not *most people*, take a few bites of your nutrition of choice. If you do find it difficult to eat right out of the water, bring some calories with you for the bike ride. At the very least, have water or a sports drink at the ready for a few swigs in the transition area. (See Chapter 9 for more information on nutrition.)

If you're starting your transition workout at a pool, a bathroom should be nearby for you to take care of your business before heading out for your ride. If the T-workout is at a lake or other body of water, be prepared to get creative. If brick-and-mortar facilities or even portable toilets are on-site, don't depend on them to be stocked and ready for you—so BYOTP. If worse comes to worse, your only option might be to find a secluded spot in a forested area. Be sure to avoid the poison ivy though!

> ### Training Tips
>
> When setting up your practice T1 (or T2), you might decide to put your hydration bottles in a fridge or cooler to keep them cool. If you do, be sure to put a big sign on your bike reminding you to get them out and on your bike before heading off.

When you're heading out for a bike ride on any average day, how do you prepare and what do you bring with you? From top to bottom, you can't ride without your helmet, sunglasses, jersey, shorts, and shoes. Do you also use socks or bike gloves? What about some sort of body lubrication? Nutritional items and supplements? Water bottle(s) or sports drinks are probably on everyone's list. If you don't have a mini-pump attached to your bike frame or a CO_2 cartridge in your bike bag, be sure you have a floor pump wherever you'll be doing the T-workout.

To Change or Not to Change?

If changing areas are available in your race, you can decide if you want to use them to change your clothes. Many people choose to change during practice workouts, but few people do so in an actual race shorter than a half-Ironman distance, which won't have designated changing areas. We recommend only changing clothes if the designated changing areas are available. If you're uncomfortable being out of the water in just a swimsuit, you can always slip some shorts or a shirt on over the suit. If you decide you're going to change your clothes when a specified area isn't available, you can "keep it clean" by wrapping a large towel around yourself (be sure it's secured!) and getting the job done.

Guys, you can perform the change by wrapping the towel around your waist and then going under the towel from below with your hands to pull your shorts down. Work the next set of shorts up under the towel until they're in place, remove the towel, and you're good to go. Ladies, you can first put on your sports bra (or the TRI top used for the event) over your swimsuit. Then work your arms out of your swimsuit straps and pull the suit down to your waist. For the bottoms, follow the same steps the guys perform. To secure the towel, you can even tuck it into your sports bra.

If you're not familiar with this trick, don't worry: you can learn it quickly. The biggest obstacle is to be sure you get a towel wide enough that when wrapped around you covers all your private spots and long enough that you can wrap it around yourself with enough extra length to tuck it in and make it secure. Some stores even sell towels specifically made for wrapping, complete with Velcro for easy securing.

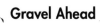 **Gravel Ahead**

Be sure to try the quick-change a few times at home before you try to rush it at a race without practice you might give everyone an intimate view of yourself in your birthday suit.

Practice Makes Perfect

When you've decided what items you'll need and what you'll be wearing for the bike, you then have to figure out how you're going to get the transition done. If you're practicing the T-workout at a public pool or lake and you have a buddy who wants to just hang out in the sun, set up your gear on the ground as you would in a real triathlon. If you're flying solo in a public place, put all your T-gear in a bag and put it in a locker or set it up in your car trunk (if it's big enough).

If you've decided you'll change after the swim, get that done first, however you decide to do it. Put on a quick coat of sunscreen, even if you had some on during your swim. Lubricate any areas you know will rub while you're on the bike. Then, double-check that your nutritional items are in place (including hydration). Put your keys in a safe spot. Some people put them in their jersey pocket (be careful they don't bounce out!); some store them in little lock boxes attached to the outside of their car; some slide the key ring over their finger and then put a glove on that hand. You could even safety-pin your keys to your waistband or something. However you choose to do it, triple-check that your keys are secure and then head out for your ride.

T1 Checklist

To help you keep track of what you need (and don't need), here's a sample race checklist:

Swim related:

❏ Towel
❏ Foot rinse supplies

Neutral:

❏ Contact solution or eye drops
❏ Transition hydration
❏ Transition snack
❏ Change of clothes
❏ First-aid kit
❏ Postworkout nutrition
❏ Sunscreen
❏ Keys/phone/cash

Bike related:

❏ Bicycle
❏ Helmet
❏ Cycling shorts
❏ Jersey or singlet
❏ Bike shoes
❏ Socks
❏ Lubrication
❏ Sunglasses
❏ Pump, CO_2, spare tube(s)
❏ Water bottles/energy drinks
❏ Bike multi-tool
❏ Floor pump
❏ Nutrition for bike segment
❏ Heart rate monitor

Some of these items are optional. Feel free to adjust the list as your experience/preference dictates.

T2: Bike to Run

T2, your second transition, is generally more straightforward than T1 because usually you have fewer things to pick up on your way out. You drop off a lot of gear but have little that you need to put on before you start the run.

Gathering Your Gear

How do you usually feel when you're finishing up a long bike ride? Maybe your legs are getting tired and your bike shorts are getting uncomfortable. Perhaps your water bottles are empty and you're *dying* of thirst. Maybe you ran out of food and you're *starving*. If it's hot outside, you might have sweat mixed with sunscreen stinging your eyes as you finish and head into transition. Make mental notes during training (and actual notes after the workouts) that will help you tailor your personal transition lists.

If the day's a scorcher, you know you'll be finishing your bike ride with sweat pouring down your body. You might want a towel handy for a quick wipe down. Even if the sweat doesn't bother you, you might want that towel to dry off before putting on some additional sunscreen. A small hand towel does the trick.

When you head out for a run, what are the essentials? Sunglasses, a jersey top, shorts, and shoes. Do you use a hat or a visor? What about socks? Do you usually lube up in certain areas? Men, do you put any sort of liquid-bandage on your nipples for protection? Be sure to pack all these things you'll use.

> **Training Tips**
>
> Even if you think you have enough to eat and drink with you on your bike, have some sort of hydration and nutrition ready for your transition time. You can't be sure how you'll feel when you're changing for the next event.

Ch-Ch-Ch-Changes

To change or not to change, that is the question (again). Some people elect to change clothes between the bike and run segment. This is rare in a race that's shorter than a half-Ironman, but it can be done. Just follow the steps we talked about in the T1 transition. Many people choose to change before a T-run while training because they're not being timed and comfort outweighs quickness. If you're comfortable running in bike shorts, keep them on and save yourself a little time.

If your bike has clipless pedals or you have specific shoes for the bike, you'll need to change into running shoes during T2. If you bike with your running shoes, you're good to go; no change is necessary in that department.

Sunglasses are another item you probably don't have to change. Unless you have a pet peeve about smudges or sweat drips on your sunglasses (which you might well acquire while on a ride), you can run with the pair you rode with. If you want a more pristine piece of eyewear, have the second set of glasses opened and ready to go.

T2 Checklist

Here's a list of what you might need for your transition. Adjust the list as your experience dictates.

Bike related:

❑ Towel   ❑ Washcloth

Neutral:

❑ Contact solution or eye drops   ❑ Transition hydration

❑ Transition snack   ❑ Change of clothes

❑ First-aid kit   ❑ Postworkout nutrition

❑ Sunscreen   ❑ Keys/phone/cash

Run related:

❑ Socks   ❑ Shoes

❑ Shorts   ❑ Jersey top

❑ Sunglasses   ❑ Hat

❑ Fuel belt   ❑ Nutrition for run

❑ Hydration for run   ❑ Lubrication/liquid bandage

No Rush, No Cry

For those triathletes who are just starting out, plan to take your time in transition, both in workouts and in races, at least at the beginning. It won't take long for you to figure out spots where you can cut time and eliminate steps from your transitions, but don't rush yourself. You'll thank us later. During workouts, try to begin your second event of a transition workout within 10 minutes of finishing the first event, but if it takes a little longer to get going, don't beat yourself up over it.

Training Tips

If you have the opportunity, go watch a TRI. Park yourself somewhere along the border of the transition area for a while, and watch the triathletes going through T1 or T2. The experience can be invaluable.

Remove everything you no longer need after coming in from one sport and then put on everything you need for the next. Take a breath. Take a drink. Grab something to eat. Recheck that you have everything you need before you head out into the great beyond.

Taking your time only adds a minute or two, whereas rushing can ruin your time in the next event. Remember the tortoise and the hare story: slow and steady wins the race (or at least gets the job done right).

The Transition Setup Challenge: Keep It Simple

By the nature of what you're trying to accomplish in transition, you might find yourself rushing things. You're going to need to keep your wits about you. To avoid making mistakes, keep things as simple as possible and set up your transition area in a way that forces you to go step by step through the gear you need to switch out.

Our favorite way to set up our transition area is to "go deep." We group all our equipment by sport and then place the equipment for each sport in order, with the things we'll put on or use first closest to where we'll be standing or sitting. The stuff we'll put on or use last goes deepest on the transition towel.

During Workouts

Logistically, you should set up your workout transition area just like you would in a race. Getting into the transition mind-set during your workouts makes it so much easier to set up your T-area during a race.

When you're planning for a transition workout, you need to be prepared ahead of time. You don't want to finish up one event and then have to spend a long time organizing yourself to go out for the next event. Get set before you start the day. We like to organize things the night before; just like before a race.

Set up your transition area using the checklists earlier in this chapter, either at home, in the trunk of your car, or wherever you'll be doing your transition. Remember, keep it simple, prepare early, and try to keep the approach similar to the one you'll have on race day.

Training Tips

If you really want to know exactly where each piece of equipment will go before you get to your race, you could divide your T-towel up into sections using a magic marker. Label each section with the item it will hold and then you won't have to worry about equipment positioning on race day.

Race Day Issues

When race day comes, you'll be prepared from all your practice. Believe in your preparation. Utilize your checklists. Bring anything you might want or might need. Once you're away from home, you've only got the goods you brought with you. However, sometimes a friend or "transition rack" acquaintance may have an extra item they're willing to share. Don't count on this, but it can happen.

One of the major differences between T-workouts and actual races is that you need to transport all your gear and your bike to the race site. Generally people utilize a backpack, duffle bag, or a specialized TRI bag to get this done. Whatever method you use, be sure you also practice packing up all your gear a couple days before the race. This helps avoid a late-night scramble the day before the race.

Most medium to large bags will probably be up to the task, as a wetsuit bag and your helmet can usually be attached to the outside of a pack. The only items you need in the bag are the smaller, more pliable items. Check it out for yourself and be sure everything fits.

On race day, remember you won't arrive, set up, and start racing immediately (unlike training). Be sure to bring any little extras you'd like to have with you before the race. Some people like to pass the time by listening to an MP3 player, reading a book, or taking a nap in the grass (don't forget to set your alarm!). If you're able to park close to the event, you might keep these prerace items in your car. If not, you can bring them to the transition area and lay them out on the towel separate from everything else. That way, they'll be at your disposal when you're setting up your T-area, and you'll be able to grab them on your way out. Extra food or drink, warm clothes, and things to keep you entertained fall into this category.

If you choose to bring along something valuable, have a plan of what you'll do with it before the race begins. Typically, race venues allow for spectators to stand just outside the transition area. You could hand off your valuables to a friend or family member to manage while you race. Or you could simply tuck it into something like a spare shoe if it's small enough, or wrap it up in your warmup clothes and leave it at your little piece of real estate marked by your towel.

Special Needs Bags

At longer races, such as the Ironman, there's typically one spot in the bike and one spot in the run where you can pick up a personally packed bag of goodies. These two special needs bags (SNBs; one for the bike, one for the run) are simple, plastic, drawstring bags that can be filled with any sort of food, drink, or supplement you want to be sure you have. Generally, triathletes fill the bags with items that aren't available from the course aid stations. After all, there's no reason to pack what's already provided for you.

The bags are usually identified with your name or race number, so volunteers can later easily match you two up. You pack the two bags at your leisure and turn them in at a special location the morning of the race. The race volunteers then take them to (or near) the midpoint of the bike and run courses where you'll pick them up during the race.

> **Coaches' Corner**
>
> We've heard of a wide array of goodies people have eaten partway through long rides or packed in their SNBs, including pretzels, potato chips, Pop-Tarts, candy bars, jelly beans, gummy candies, energy drinks, and a specific soda pop or other drink. Is your special treat on that list? What else would you add?

What to Bring

Some people don't think an SNB will be that useful or helpful. Don't underestimate the power of the SNB! Throughout your training, there must have been at least one time when you started to crave some specific item while you were out for a workout. Maybe you felt like if you didn't get that special candy or drink soon, you wouldn't be able to survive for another half mile. Perhaps you then stopped at a gas station and picked up that special something and it made you feel like a million bucks. Think about it. What was that special something you needed?

Don't only think about food and drink for your special needs bags. Bring all the supplements you'll need for the bike as you come out of the bike transition; likewise for the run. It's a great idea to put some backup supplements in your special needs bags, too. That way, if you accidentally drop, lose, or destroy some supplements along the way, you'll be able to replenish your supply at the special needs stop. Also include any medicine or extra gear you might need during the day.

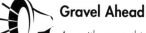

Gravel Ahead

As with everything on race day, don't try anything new with your SNB. Pack food, drinks, and supplements you know have worked in the past. Don't put some random treats in there because you hear at the last minute how well something worked for someone else.

Logistics

You'll be packing these bags up on the night before race day or the morning of, and generally speaking, once you hand them off to race officials, the bags won't be refrigerated during transportation or out on the course. Keep that in mind. If your race is in a hot climate, don't throw a chocolate candy bar in your run bag without something to keep it cool. Especially in an Ironman, you probably won't be halfway through the run portion of the race until mid-afternoon or later … and the sun will have turned your treat into a mess!

Some people try to insulate their goodies with some sort of wrapping and maybe an icepack or two. Sealable bags do a great job keeping your dry treats dry. You might also want to freeze any drinks and candy bars the night before. After several hours in the heat, even a bottle filled with one giant ice cube will melt. By the time you get to it, it probably won't be cold … but hopefully it won't be boiling hot, either.

Training Tips

Don't forget that water expands when it freezes, so be sure there's room for that expansion when you stick a bottle in the freezer. You don't want to wake up, open the freezer, and find an exploded mess.

Most people pack their SNBs the night before the race (or even earlier). If you put them in the refrigerator or freezer the night before the race, you might want to put a note on the door saying "Don't forget SNBs!"

The Process

When you head over to the race venue, you'll drop off your two SNBs at the designated spot. You'll probably be able to spot the area by the rather long procession of people, slowly moving forward in the dark of the early morning. If the line looks huge, don't panic! It's normally a quick drop, and they'll get you through in time.

After you hand over the SNBs to the race crew, they transport the bags to the right spot on the course and arrange them in numerical order. When you start to get close to the special needs area, either a volunteer calls out your number to another who gets your bag for you, or you'll use well-marked signs to help pinpoint your bag's location.

> ### Coaches' Corner
>
> Depending on the setup, you might need to drop your bike SNB with one race official and your run SNB with another. Or you might just hand them off to a single person. Whatever the setup, the race volunteers will be able to guide you.

Once you have your SNB in hand, you can slow down (or stop all together) to grab what you want and drop what you don't. Some efficient triathletes can grab their bag and continue without slowing their pace, but that can be very difficult. Especially if it's your first time, don't rush yourself. Get everything arranged exactly like you want it before getting back into race mode.

> ### Gravel Ahead
>
> Depending on the race/situation, you might not get your SNBs back. Don't put anything in an SNB that you absolutely want to have after the race is done. Pack your bag with items you *might* want during the race but you won't miss if you never see them again. The main goal of the special needs volunteers is to get your bag to you during the race. Expect to get nothing back, and you won't be disappointed.

Your transitions aren't black box mysteries. Through practice and perseverance, you'll figure out how best to set up your transition area and go through the steps … and you'll be successful. Have fun with all the planning, practice, and strategy involved.

The Least You Need to Know

◆ Practicing your transitions will make you successful on race day.

◆ With a solid checklist to go by, gathering your transition gear should be a no-brainer.

◆ Although you'll be excited, try not to rush yourself in transition; instead, go step by step through the process.

Part  Beyond the Four Disciplines of Triathlon

Swimming, biking, running, and transitions are the tangible elements of triathlon from the time the gun goes off until you cross the finish line. However, you need to factor several other aspects into your program both during training and racing. Some people choose to "wing it" when it comes to these extras, and that may cause problems, both immediately and later down the road.

Nutrition is an essential part of the sport of triathlon, both during training and races. It can make the difference between walking and running, "bonking" and finishing with a smile. Weight training and stretching are two other often-overlooked aspects of this multisport. We explain all this completely.

And perhaps the most problematic part of triathlon is making sure you get enough rest. Even the most elite athletes—who know their bodies need time to recover and absorb all the hard training they're doing—blow off resting. You won't fall into the trap of feeling like you need to work out all the time, because we'll be there to guide you.

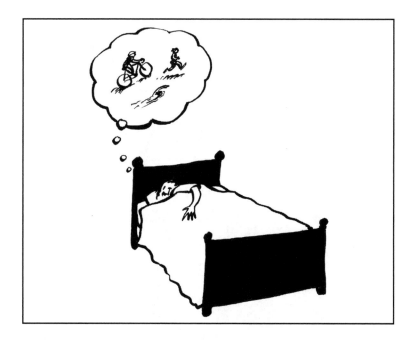

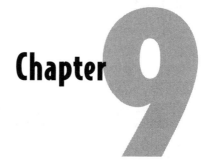

Chapter 9

Fueling Up

In This Chapter

- ◆ The makeup of essential nutrients
- ◆ The role of fuel before, during, and following activity
- ◆ What carries well on the fly
- ◆ Understanding ergogenic aids

It's important to understand how diet and the sport of triathlon are connected. During training, racing, and recovery, your body relies on essential nutrients to keep you going. To optimize your body's performance, you need to learn how your body reacts to different fueling options while following some key nutritional guidelines.

Although we can and do give you guidance in this chapter, we can't give you a cut-and-dry "this is what you should do" fueling rule to follow, because what works for one person won't necessarily work for someone else. Experiment with various preworkout meals and different fueling options during your training. In the weeks before your race, you'll have plenty of opportunities to try many different techniques, theories, or combinations of foods. Keeping track of how your body reacts to each helps you plan your nutrition in the future.

Filling Your Tank with High Octane

In the early days of triathlon and other endurance sports, little was known about fueling the body. Soda and fast food were as acceptable as oatmeal and bananas. Now, many years later, we've learned a lot more about what it takes to efficiently run the human body, and nutrition has become as important as proper training.

Coaches' Corner

One of our TRI mentors, Bob Babbitt, competed in the Hawaii Ironman in its third year (1980). Back then, as a medical precaution, athletes were required to weigh in at checkpoints on the run course. Anyone who lost 5 percent of his or her body weight was pulled out of the race. Bob was prepared for a long day in the sun and had brought several loaves of Hawaiian sweet bread with him. He "fueled up" at very regular intervals. At the second run checkpoint, race officials were shocked to find that Bob was *gaining* weight! Talk about carbo-loading!

When you think about nutrition, it's important to understand the basic principles. Our bodies need six different kinds of nutrients to function properly:

◆ Water   ◆ Protein

◆ Carbohydrates   ◆ Vitamins

◆ Fats   ◆ Minerals

Our bodies are about 60 to 70 percent water, and when we don't take in enough H_2O throughout the day, we get dehydrated. This causes a reduction in our blood plasma, which in turn forces the heart to work harder. The bottom line: performance is negatively impacted. Adults should consume between 1 and 1.5 milliliters of water for each calorie spent in the day. For example, a person who expends 2,000 calories a day should consume 2 or 3 liters.

Carbohydrates (*carbo* means "carbon," and *hydrate* means "water") come in two main groups: simple (sugars) and complex (starches/fiber). Glucose is the preferred fuel for most of the body's functions. It's especially important for fueling the brain and nervous system, which is almost exclusively dependent on glucose for energy. In general, carbohydrates are an integral part of training, racing, and our overall diet. Approximately 50 percent of your total calories should come from carbohydrates.

Coaches' Corner

Olive oil is a great source of monounsaturated fat. Extra-virgin olive oil has a higher level of free radical–fighting vitamin E than "regular" olive oil. It has been linked to lower rates of heart disease, colon cancer, diabetes, and osteoporosis. And it tastes good to boot! Toss in a little with balsamic vinegar for a quick salad dressing.

Fats are an important component in the diet. Nutritionally speaking, fat provides a concentrated energy source (9 calories per gram). Fats are also a source of essential fatty acids, which the body needs but does not produce in sufficient quantities. Fat comes in "good" and "bad" varieties. *Unsaturated fats* (monounsaturated and polyunsaturated) are better for you than *saturated fats*, which are linked to higher risks of cardiovascular disease.

One fat to avoid: trans-fatty acid. This manufactured health risk is created when polyunsaturated oils are hydrogenated, resulting in fatty acids with unusual shapes. Read food labels and stay clear of transfats or "partially hydrogenated" oils. Approximately 30 percent of total calories should come from fat with a focus on unsaturated.

Protein is made up of amino acids, of which there are about 20 kinds that we need to function properly. The body makes about half of these, and the others come from our diet and are called *essential amino acids*. Protein can be used as a fuel (4 calories per gram); however, it's typically more involved in recovery and building new tissues. Plus, protein helps carry oxygen, as a component of hemoglobin. Approximately 20 percent of your total calories should come from protein.

Vitamins are *organic* compounds that are vital to life and can be divided into two main groups: fat soluble (vitamins A, D, E, and K) and water soluble (B vitamins and C). Fat soluble vitamins are absorbed into the lymph (lymphatic tissue), can travel on protein carriers in the blood, and can be stored in fatty tissues. You must be careful not to consume an excess of A, D, E, or K because they can build to toxic concentrations. This should not be an issue for those who eat a balanced diet with some supplementation. It's more a risk for those who do extreme supplementation of these vitamins. Water soluble vitamins on the other hand are not stored. They are absorbed into the bloodstream and processed, and excess amounts pass out of the body through the urine.

Minerals are naturally occurring *inorganic* (without carbon) elements and fall into two categories: major minerals and trace minerals. Some of the major minerals include calcium, phosphorus, potassium, and sodium. Some of the trace minerals include iron, manganese, copper, and iodine.

Putting It All Together

Our bodies rely on carbohydrates, fats, and protein for energy, with carbohydrates as the preferred source because its energy is easily released and used by our bodies. During low- to moderate-intensity activity, we use both glucose (glycogen—a stored form of glucose) and fatty acids for fuel.

When you keep your system in the aerobic zone, your body uses glucose and fat as energy. When you increase the intensity, your body shifts away from fatty acids, and glucose becomes the sole fuel.

> **Training Tips**
>
> Glycogen depletion can also occur during repeated short, high-intensity workouts such as interval training or hill repeats. Keep in the aerobic zone as much as possible, and take in more calories through food and drink.

But you have only a limited store of glucose available in your body, and your brain and nervous system need glucose and have first dibs on what's in your blood. When your body is in glycogen-only mode and you're training for long periods of time, at high intensities, or both, you can be burning upward of 600 to 800 calories per hour. The only way to maintain your glucose stores is by diet.

No Meat? No Dairy? No Problem!

Before we move onto the more conventional discussion about nutrition, it's worth mentioning that you can be a triathlete *and* a vegetarian (no meat products) or vegan (no animal products including dairy and eggs) at the same time. People have done it in the past, and people are going to continue to do it in the future. Like becoming a vegetarian in normal life, becoming a vegetarian triathlete forces a little more time and research than an active omnivore. Vegan triathletes have to be even a little more focused.

Eating as a vegetarian or vegan can be relatively straightforward if you're doing the shopping and preparation of your food. The difficulty may arise if you want to use meal replacement product or other manufactured nutritional supplement. Because there are so many technical names for different animal based ingredients (and more seem to be created every day), we won't even try to list them here. Our recommendation is to use online search engines to find discussion boards or other websites where you can benefit from people who have already done the research.

Some supplements have been created purposefully with only vegetarian ingredients and a few with only vegan ingredients. If you see a product but cannot decipher if it's vegetarian or vegan, one easy way to find out is to contact the manufacturer. Most products have 800 numbers or e-mail addresses you can use to contact the customer service department with questions.

> ### Coaches' Corner
>
> Colin did his first Ironman as an omnivore. He ate anything he could get his hands on—steak, burgers, chicken, turkey, etc. All were fair game on a daily basis. He felt great during training and during his race. About a year before his second Ironman, he decided to try to become a vegetarian. It presented some challenges at first, but he adapted to the lifestyle. Again, he felt great during training and during his race. No matter what your special nutritional needs are (whether by choice or genetics), you can succeed at triathlon!

Preworkout Chow

Never work out on an empty stomach. *But*, you might be thinking, *as a kid I was told to not go swimming until X minutes after I ate.* Find a middle ground. Don't eat a large, greasy meal just before working out, but eat something. When training, your body is burning calorie after calorie. If you've had no food recently, you might feel like a car running on fumes. Always try to have some sort of small nutritious meal before your workout.

The exact amount of time needed between eating and working out varies from person to person. It also depends on the workout or race you're about to do. The first time you plan on eating before a workout, try it a couple hours out from your workout. If it goes well, try nudging your meal closer to your exercise start time. The goal is to have your stomach feeling comfortable and not hungry when you begin.

What's for Breakfast?

Most people who work out in the morning usually do so right after waking up. Many people do this every day and feel like it works fine for them. There are two possible problems with this method:

♦ Glycogen (stores of glucose) levels are low.

♦ Hydration levels are low, and dehydration is a risk.

Remember, it's been 12 or so hours since your last meal (depending on your sleeping and eating schedules). If your body has low amounts of calories to fuel the workout, you may feel lethargic and won't get as much out of the training/racing.

You have several options for early morning preworkout chow. Most nutritionists recommend a meal that includes carbohydrates, fat, and protein, with the bulk of the calories coming from carbohydrates. Including some protein and fat helps keep you feeling full longer and contributes to the gradual release of energy into the body. Try to keep fat and protein calorie intake to approximately 15 percent of your total meal. If you consume too much, it will slow digestion and absorption of the fuel. Work with different pretraining/prerace meals to find what works best and agrees with you.

Here are some breakfast options popular among the triathletes we know:

♦ Well-balanced nutrition bar

♦ Banana and yogurt

♦ Peanut butter on toast, English muffin, or bagel

♦ Cereal or oatmeal with protein powder

♦ Frozen fruit and yogurt smoothie

Training Tips

If you have to start working out the minute you wake up because your schedule absolutely does not permit any other option, then at a minimum, take a big drink of water or sports drink before you start moving.

A nutrition bar is the quickest option and doesn't take any concentration in the morning. The other foods are pretty easy as well. You can find protein powder at any general nutrition store in several flavors. If you have food allergies, check the ingredients in these powders, as most contain soy. If you're lactose intolerant, steer clear of the whey powders derived from dairy sources. Some of the other types include egg, egg/milk, and rice bases. As with any nutritional supplements, check the labels and give a little more consideration to powders with natural ingredients. The instructions on the container will explain how to make a protein shake by

Coaches' Corner

Yogurt, especially fruit yogurt, has a good balance of carbohydrates and protein, which contribute to energy during workouts, exercise recovery, and muscle growth. Plus, yogurt is a good source of conjugated linoleic acid, an essential polyunsaturated fatty acid *not* made within the body. So eat up!

mixing a certain amount of the powder with water or milk. That works, but we prefer to just throw a little powder onto other types of food to give it a protein kick.

Experiment with some or all of these food options. Try to keep track of what you eat before your workouts and note how you felt. Hopefully you felt great the entire workout after one of these suggested meals. But maybe you got hungry as soon as you started working out. Did you get a cramp? Did you have to use the bathroom in a bad way? Keeping track of what works and what doesn't helps you plan your future preworkout meals and will be invaluable when deciding what to eat on the morning of your race.

Fueling During the Day

If you're planning a training session in the afternoon or after work, try to be conscious of what you eat for lunch or your midday snack. Avoid the greases. Avoid the extreme fats and oils. In general, follow the breakfast guidelines listed earlier. Eat smart, and get some good carbohydrates, fat, and protein.

If you're going out for a long ride and don't want to worry about finding a restroom, avoid foods high in fiber and fructose (sugar) such as whole-wheat products, bran cereals, fruits, vegetables, juices, energy bars, and some sports drinks, which can cause diarrhea and other stomach discomfort for some people. Read the label. If fructose appears early on the list of ingredients, be forewarned. Experiment and see what works for you. (If you don't have trouble with this, go for it.)

Eating on the Move

Fueling up while on the move is both an art and a science that you really need to practice. Obviously, you're not able to consume anything during the swim. Hopefully you're not drinking much water, because the only source would be the lake or ocean! When you're out of the water, you'll ease into your nutrition plan.

Out of the three disciplines, the bike is probably the most important regarding "eating on the move." It's the longest segment so you have plenty of time, and your upper body is relatively motionless (compared with running). You can clip through the miles and replenish calories lost in the swim, those you're burning on the bike, and pack a little reserve of calories for the run.

Many people like to pack their nutrition bars, gels, and supplements in their jersey pockets. Some use a Bento box Velcroed to the frame (top tube) of their bike. We've seen triathletes duct tape the top of gel packets to the frame. When they need one, they pull off the packet. The duct tape holds the top portion on the frame. We've seen others

Gravel Ahead

After a tough swim, food might not want to settle very easily. You might not have any trouble, but be cautious in the transition after a swim. Give your body a chance to acclimate from horizontal swimming to a completely different movement.

Training Tips

One hand near the stem offers more steering stability while you're negotiating your nutrition.

unwrap energy bars and press them on their handle bars, stem, and frame using the bar's own sticky quality. If you're in a race or just don't like dealing with opening packaging, you can precut bar packages prior to a ride.

You have a lot of options, so use what works best for you. Practice many different systems and figure out what you're most comfortable with. You have to be able to take in nutrition while maintaining a straight pace line, and avoiding pitfalls, competitors, friends, or vehicles on the road. If you need to, slow down while you fuel. You can simply coast, keep an eye on the road, steer, and slowly ingest the food or drink.

You can also take in fuel on the run if the distance you're going warrants it. For example, if you're out on a short training run or in a sprint-distance TRI, you might not need to replenish your calories before you finish. However, if you're out on a long run or in an Ironman, you'll need to fuel up during the run. It's more difficult for most people to eat during the run, so you'll really need to learn what works for you. While your stomach is bouncing down the road with you, it's difficult to digest and absorb nutrients.

One thing that works for us is to spread out many small portions of food. For example, you could take a small bite of an energy bar, take your time to chew it up, and follow it up with a baby sip of water or sports drink. This is easier on your digestive system than scarfing down a full bar all at once. Some athletes choose to avoid "solid" foods all together on the run and use only gels. The same concept holds true with gels as with solid food: take a little at a time.

It's critical to make notes after a training session on your nutrition strategy. When you find what agrees with you, you'll be that much closer to getting to the finish line with a smile.

Liquids vs. Solids

There's no one way to tackle a nutrition plan. We know triathletes who prefer liquids only, gels only, or solids only, and we know some who mix the three. Just like practicing a good overall diet, we recommend variety.

How can you train and race with liquids only? It depends somewhat on the distance you're training for. If you're getting ready for a shorter distance race and your workouts aren't draining your energy stores, perhaps you can get by on water or a sports drink. There are also products you can add to water or a sports drink that contain pure carbohydrate calories. Some of these powders are tasteless and provide a whopping 100 calories per scoop. The best part is that these powders are very water-soluble, so you can add several scoops to one water bottle. You can easily head out on a ride with two full bottles and have enough energy to carry you for hours.

Between liquids and solids are gels. Gels typically come in a pliable packet. You simply tear off the top and squeeze the gel into your mouth. It might seem strange or gross to get your calories like this, but give it a try. Gels come in tons of different flavors. Don't be overwhelmed by the wide assortment of options; just keep your mind open and give your taste buds and stomach a variety of possibilities. Find a few you like and rotate them.

Training Tips

Ladies, you can stick 3 or 4 packets in your sports bra. It isn't too uncomfortable, and you don't have to worry about carrying a flask (which also allows you to keep a variety of flavors). This is better for shorter distance rides and races.

If you don't like carrying several gel packets to get you through a longer run, you might want to look into using a gel flask. This plastic container is like a mini-water bottle that holds the contents of three to five gel packets and can be carried on a run or Velcroed to your bike frame. It's a good idea to add a couple ounces of water into your flask before adding the gels. Then shake it up a bit after the gel is in there. This helps thin the contents and makes it easier to squeeze it out (most gels are on the thick side).

Check out the ingredients in gels. Some offer longer chained glucose, which are released into the bloodstream more slowly. This may be better for longer durations as it doesn't spike your blood sugar levels as quickly. It's a good idea to read up on the different types of gels and what's inside before you make a purchase.

Solids, as you might guess, are anything from energy bars, candy bars, Pop-Tarts, fig bars, pretzels, crackers, bananas and other fruits … the list goes on and on. You have many options here.

A side note on energy bars: not all are created equal. You might want to do a little research and find a bar that contains natural ingredients. Try avoiding those with too many chemicals, preservatives, and transfats listed on the label. If you don't know what an ingredient is, look it up. Learn about what you're putting in your body. Ideally, you'll find something that not only tastes good but is also packed with nutrients.

Experiment with fuel sources in different temperatures both on the bike and the run. You might find that liquids and gels work best for you on the run while you prefer solids and liquids on the bike. When training in really hot temperatures, you might stay away from solids all together. Your body will tell you what best works for you! When you're training and racing for longer distances, eat and drink early and often. In a TRI race, you might have to ease into eating after the swim, but then it's important to get on some kind of a schedule (depending on the distance). For example, you might want to set your sports watch to beep every 15 minutes to remind you to take a swig or bite.

Salty Dog

Sodium is a critical electrolyte in the human body and is especially important during any long or hot workouts or races. In these conditions most experienced athletes supplement with sodium to help manage fluid levels (hydration) and electrolyte balance. You lose both fluids and electrolytes through sweat. It's not uncommon to lose 1 or 2 quarts of fluid during an hour or so of training in hot and humid conditions. If you don't replace this loss, you could find yourself dehydrated very quickly. This results in a reduction in performance and, if not dealt with, could lead to heat-related illness. On the other end of the fluid/electrolyte balance is overhydration. If you drink too much water, you can dilute the sodium content in your blood. Sodium also assists in moving fluid from the stomach to the bloodstream.

You can ingest sodium in different ways, including some sports drinks, salt tablets (small pills made up of sodium), or buffered salt tablets (which are high in sodium but also include other nutrients like calcium, magnesium, potassium, and zinc). The collection of minerals in buffered salt tablets work together to help reduce the risk of muscle cramps, heat fatigue, and *hyponatremia*. For some, the buffered versions are easier to digest. Steve uses a plastic tube filled with the tablets during long rides and runs; Colin seals his up in a resealable plastic bag.

Gravel Ahead

If you're interested in experimenting with sodium supplementation, we recommend you first talk with your doctor.

def•i•ni•tion

Low blood sodium levels, or **hyponatremia,** can occur from ingesting too little sodium or too much water and can be a serious health threat if not managed promptly. Some symptoms include nausea, apathy, confusion, and fatigue. Sodium intake needs to be more scrutinized during high-intensity activity and under hot conditions. Experiment with different ways to increase sodium intake during training and races.

Race-Fueling Specifics

Fueling during a race is similar to fueling during training, except some races have aid stations on the bike and run courses that give you hydration and nutrition. That means less for you to carry! Depending on the race venue and distance, aid stations can be spread out every few miles. For example, the last Olympic-distance race Steve did had an aid station upon exiting T1, two out on the bike course, and one every 2 miles on the run course. Be aware that shorter races might not offer any aid stations at all. Verify the race layout prior to the race using a website or literature you receive in the mail.

Grabbing food and drink from an aid station can be a bit of a challenge. It's not as much of an issue while running: you simply slow down and take the offering from a volunteer. They usually do a good job announcing if they have water, a sports drink, or some sort of food. Sometimes the station also has signs that indicate what you can get where.

When you're cruising along toward an aid station and you reach out for some nutrition, don't keep a rigid arm or hand; let your arm sway back a little to cushion the transfer. Let's say you're attempting for a sports drink bottle. Slow down, point to the volunteer so they know you're interested, and grab the bottle, remembering to let your arm sway back upon "impact." It might take a couple tries to get it. We suggest you practice this at home with a friend or family member.

Gravel Ahead

Beyond verifying where and how many aid stations are available at the race, be sure to find out *what* will be served. The nutrition that works for you might not be offered. If you feel most comfortable using a specific gel that's not provided, bring your own.

Recovery Dining

The calories and sugars you took in during the workout were to keep you moving forward and feed your brain and nervous system. When you're done with a long or intense workout, your muscles are empty. Filling your tank up promptly contributes to a quick recovery and ensures you're at your best for the next workout.

After a long workout or crossing the finish line, focus on replenishing your fluids. Drink water or a fluid replacement sports drink. This becomes more important if you feel you've neglected it during the activity. Next, replenish your glycogen stores. Eat something with a carbohydrate focus within the first hour. Ideally, you should do this within the first 30 minutes (the sooner the better). This is the best time to expedite your recovery.

Training Tips

If you can stomach a pint of chocolate milk after a workout or race, go for it. This has been dubbed as one of the best recovery fuels because it has the right balance of carbohydrates, fat, and protein.

The type of carbohydrates you eat to recover is important. Simple carbohydrates raise glucose and insulin levels the fastest. So grab an apple before a bowl of spaghetti. When simple carbs are readily available in the blood, movement of glucose into muscle cells is swift and glycogen stores build more quickly. Why the haste? Muscle cells are most ready to absorb replenishments of glucose soon after exercise. Some call it a calorie window of opportunity or carbohydrate window. As time passes after a workout, the cells' resistance to glucose and insulin temporarily goes up, making recovery more of a challenge.

In addition to the glucose focus, small amounts of protein have been found to aid the insulin response and, hence, contribute to recovery. The debate about the exact amount has not yet been settled. Some suggest a 4-to-1 carbohydrates to protein ratio. If you ingest too much, it slows the stomach from emptying. Keep drinking fluids, and be sure you eat a well-balanced meal with protein, fat, and carbohydrates later that day.

Reward Meals

The very thought of a reward meal brings a smile to any athlete's face. The concept is simple: treat yourself to something you love following a tough workout, a milestone in your TRI training, a first race, or a new PR (personal record), whatever the reason may be and whatever the treat may be. We know triathletes who use ice cream, chocolate, Krispy Kreme donuts, or a bag of fries as their treats. The point is to set little goals and milestones and reward yourself for meeting them.

Reward meals give you something extra to look forward to and add to the overall fun of the sport. Don't take it too seriously. Have fun and enjoy the journey—knowing a treat is waiting for you!

Coaches' Corner

When training for his first Ironman, Colin decided he'd reward himself after every long ride/T-run with a frozen pizza and a beer. Post workout, he'd have a banana and an energy bar, followed by a well-balanced (and large) meal. For dinner that night, "healthy" went by the wayside as he cooked a pizza and cracked open a beer. Why frozen? He's just loved frozen pizzas since he was a kid. Whenever he was out riding for several hours on end, he always knew he'd have his frozen pizza later that night. It really kept him going. What is your ideal reward meal?

Ergogenic Aids

Ergo ... *what?* No, we're not going to tell you how to position yourself at your computer desk to avoid carpal tunnel. Ergogenic aids are anything that improves (or is thought to improve) one's performance (*ergo* means "work"; *genic* means "gives rise to"). It could be a specific flavor energy gel, a secret smoothie concoction you make up, or taking a whiff of peppermint essential oil before a race. For our purposes here, we focus on food supplements.

 Training Tips _____

Sports drinks vary in carbohydrate concentration, with the average range between 6 and 8 percent. A concentration below 5 percent might not give you the energy required for optimal performance, and a concentration of 10 percent or more might impair absorption. Check the label.

Caffeine

Let's start with perhaps one of the most widely used ergogenic aids in existence: caffeine, in the form of coffee, tea, cola, energy drinks, chocolate, caffeine tablets, and more. The findings are across the board regarding caffeine; for every article you read about how wonderful it is, you can find an article that says the exact opposite, so be careful experimenting with caffeine.

Caffeine has been shown to lower perceived exertion. In other words, you could maintain a higher intensity without feeling like you were pushing it. Caffeine is also purported to help conserve the body's glycogen levels, allowing for longer and more intense efforts.

Caffeine is a diuretic, which means it will probably make you have to go to the bathroom more often. Therefore, maintaining proper hydration and electrolyte balance becomes more of a challenge.

Coaches' Corner

The effects of caffeine are directly proportional to tolerance. If you're not a coffee drinker and have a cup prior to a workout, the effects will be greater than if you drink a cup every morning.

One more caveat: some TRI governing bodies such as the USA Triathlon and International Olympic Committee have ruled high levels of caffeine illegal for competition. However, the levels are extreme. You would have to drink about 8 (5-ounce) cups of coffee in an hour to reach the illegal threshold.

Glucosamine

Glucosamine is a supplement associated with improved joint function. Some studies have found that it can alleviate the symptoms of arthritis; others say it can contribute to the lubrication around joints. It really depends on what you read and who you talk to. In our experience, we've seen some benefits using this product when running mileage goes up. Give it a try if you have some joint pain. The two camps of scientists either say "it helps" or "it doesn't help." As far as we know, there aren't any studies that say glucosamine could have adverse affects.

Glutamine

Glutamine is a naturally occurring substance in the body that has been linked with many benefits such as muscle growth and recovery, improved insulin metabolism, and immune system support due to its ability to improve glucose absorption. There is no definitive evidence that taking glutamine supplements will positively impact your performance. Again, if you are interested in this ergogenic aid, we recommend additional research.

Creatine

Creatine is a certain blend of protein (amino acids) in the body that can be part of the energy release at maximal exertion that lasts only a few seconds. Some people believe that taking creatine supplements can aid in recovery and enhance strength. The science is still out on this topic. However, most studies suggest that if creatine supplements do have a positive impact, they're best suited for short burst of power activities and not muscular endurance. If you decide to try creatine, we suggest you do some further research first to better understand its affects on the body.

Be warned that the U.S. Food and Drug Administration (FDA) has received several complaints from people who have used creatine and had negative side affects. Many scientists advise against its use.

More Ergogenics

You can find many other ergogenic aids on the market, including the following:

- Choline
- Chromium
- Branched-chain amino acids (BCAA)
- Medium chain triglycerides (MCT)
- Sodium phosphate
- Glycerol

We are avid believers in keeping things simple, especially when starting out. If you need an energy boost, try some caffeine. If your knees are bugging you, try some glucosamine. If you're just starting out or just doing TRI for fun and personal accomplishment, you probably don't want to worry about some of the more unproven aids. If you do decide you want to try some of the more risky ergogenic aids, do some serious research about how these can impact your body, and talk to your doctor.

For most ergogenic aids you'll find contradicting reports, insufficient studies, and questions about long-term effects. Many of the supplements out there are just that—supplements. You can meet most of your nutritional requirements naturally through diet. For example, creatine can be found in both meat and fish.

When using ergogenic aids, be sure to keep within recommended doses. Furthermore, there may be potential issues associated with mixing ergogenic aids. We recommend you have an in-depth conversation with your health-care provider if you're interested in pursuing them further.

Nutrition is a key part of TRI. How you decide to apply it directly impacts your experience. Successful TRI nutrition is based on the timing, the type, and the quality of the fuel you consume.

> **Gravel Ahead**
>
> The supplement industry is not heavily regulated, and these products do not have to go through any FDA approval. Product purity and quality are not necessarily monitored or controlled. If you're using supplements, be sure you go with a reputable company that you trust. See if your physician can point you in the right direction.

The Least You Need to Know

- Carbohydrates and fat are the body's two main sources of energy.

- Experiment with different food strategies during training to find what works best for you.

- Stay on top of your hydration; drink early and often.

- Fill up on simple carbohydrates soon after exercise to aid in recovery.

- Research and tread carefully when deciding whether or not to try an ergogenic aid.

10

Flex and Flexibility

In This Chapter

◆ Why we lift, why we stretch

◆ What makes up a weight training program

◆ Understanding how it all fits

◆ Suggested exercises and stretches

Strength and flexibility training play an important role in overall triathlon conditioning (preparing your body for TRI through exercising, diet, and mental preparation). Practicing consistent strength training and stretching programs both improves your overall experience and reduces your chance of injury. In this chapter, you learn some key movements with a strong focus on proper technique, as incorrect technique could lead to injury.

Weight Training 101

Being "fit" requires cardiovascular fitness, muscular strength, muscular endurance, flexibility, and a balanced body composition. Your TRI training naturally contributes to many of these components. However, adding a supplemental weight training program enhances overall fitness gains. Generally, weight training (a.k.a. resistance training) has been associated with improving strength, bone density, and overall TRI performance. Possibly the most important benefit associated with weight training is that it reduces your risk of injury.

Coaches' Corner

One of the greatest challenges triathletes face at the beginning of training is muscular conditioning. Riding a bike can cause aches and pains in many areas that may have nothing to do with TRI- or bike-specific condition (or lack thereof). Your neck and shoulder muscles might get tight or sore, your triceps might burn from holding yourself up, and your lower back might hurt. You can reduce these common symptoms by adhering to a regular resistance training program. The stronger you are throughout your body, the better you'll be able to cope with what transpires from the sport of TRI.

Like with any hard swim/bike/run sessions, the first step involved in any resistance session is the warm-up. You can warm up with a low-level aerobic activity such as walking, cycling, or beginning the workout session with a light set for about 10 minutes. The objective is to gradually increase your heart rate, blood pressure, oxygen consumption, and muscle elasticity— in other words, get your body ready for some action. Skipping this step throws the rest of the workout out of sync.

As with your hard aerobic sessions, each lifting session should include a cool-down. You can do the same activities as you did before the workout session or mix things up. Just slow things down for 10 minutes or so. The objective is to gradually decrease your heart rate, blood pressure, and help process/redistribute postexercise hormones and lactic acid.

The main workout session entails repetitions (*reps*) and *set(s)*. Laying on your back on a weight bench, holding a barbell above your chest with both hands, bringing it down to your chest and pushing it back up is a single bench press rep. We recommend performing 8 to 12 reps for most of the exercises in our program; that's a set. For example, 8 pull-ups constitutes a set. Completing 1 set of 8 to 12 reps of 12 different exercises represents completing one *circuit*.

def•i•ni•tion

Reps are simply individual movements. A **set** is a group of reps. Reps and sets build with a series of different exercises to produce a **circuit**. **Load** is the amount of weight you use. **Tempo** (coming up in a few paragraphs) is the speed at which you conduct a movement or exercise.

The *load*, or amount of weight you use for each exercise, depends on where you are in the program. We recommend starting out gradually to allow your body a chance to condition itself. Keep the weight light and the number of reps on the higher end of the 8 to 12 range. The best way to determine the right load is by trial and error. Do your best to hypothesize a weight you can do 8 to 12 times with good form. If your hunch is off, make the necessary adjustments.

The goal in TRI resistance training varies depending on what part of the program you're in. In the prep and build phases, the goal is to increase strength. During the peak phase, you'll just want to maintain your strength.

Next we look at *tempo*. There are two phases: the work, or shortening (*concentric*) and the return to its resting state, or lengthening (*eccentric*). For example, in a biceps curl, the concentric phase occurs when you lift up the weight; the eccentric phase occurs as you lower it. Many people focus on or think only about the work portion of a movement. However, the lengthening component is just as, if not more, important. The recommended tempo is 1 or 2 seconds concentric and 2 to 4 seconds eccentric. If you need to, count out loud during your movements until you get the rhythm down.

Opinions differ on how much rest you should take between sets. Some say rest as you need it, with less at the beginning and more toward the end of a workout. Others say to use a range of 30 to 120 seconds between sets for a moderate resistance training program. See what feels right for you, probably somewhere in the middle. The amount of rest you require between sets depends not only on where you are in your workout but also on how heavy you're lifting.

We've already looked at *frequency*, *intensity*, and *time* (duration) from an aerobic TRI perspective (see Chapter 4). Conceptually, it's the same for resistance training. Here we'll also add *type*, including free weights, machines, body weight, elastic bands, etc.

> **Coaches' Corner**
>
> Muscle trivia! You have approximately 650 muscles in your body. The largest is the *latissimus dorsi*, which runs along the side and middle of your back. It contributes in swimming during the pull and roll. The strongest muscle in the body is the *gluteus maximus* (a.k.a. the butt). It comes in handy during the bike, especially when climbing hills.

> **def•i•ni•tion**
>
> How many days a week you work out is the **frequency**. **Intensity** is a combination of the reps/sets/load. **Time** (duration) is what your watch says but also how many exercises are performed. **Type** is the activity of resistance training.

Why Do It?

Why should you incorporate resistance training into your TRI program? The simple and fast answer is: it makes you stronger. The stronger and more conditioned you are, the better you'll be able to adapt to and progress in the sport of TRI. Resistance training also improves time to exhaustion or the level at which you fatigue. This is critical to TRI, especially as the distance of training/racing increases.

Resistance training has also been linked to tolerance and blood lactate levels. Like specific TRI training, working with resistance over time has been shown to reduce lactate concentration in blood (at the same workloads) as well as increase one's threshold or tolerance of lactic acid. Simply put, time spent resistance training helps prevent that burning feeling in your muscles caused by lactate.

Moreover, weight training has been connected with improved bone density (*mucho importante* as we age) and reduced chance of injury. The impact provided by resistance training has a way of galvanizing our bones unlike any other mode of exercise. Resistance training is regularly prescribed as a method to treat and prevent *osteoporosis*.

Besides strengthening body components, weight training can also reduce your chances of injury by creating balance and symmetry. Lack of symmetry is one of the leading causes of injury. For example, if your front leg muscles (quadriceps) and back leg muscles (hamstrings) are way out of balance, you'd be at greater risk of injury. The same goes for the outer and inner leg muscles ... or any set of counterbalanced muscles. When one area is forced to pick up slack from other regions, it can overwork itself or nearby connective tissues.

def•i•ni•tion

Osteoporosis is a disease in which the bones become extremely porous, more susceptible to fracture, and heal more slowly.

When Do I Do It?

The question of when to weight train is an interesting one in conjunction with TRI. Some experts believe that all triathletes must incorporate resistance training into their weekly programs. Others think it should be optional and that time is better spent in TRI specific training (especially for beginners). We see a middle ground. Many other variables come into play such as age, gender, prior strength training experience, and time to train.

One rule of thumb when it comes to age is the 30-year cut-off. Triathletes under 30 years old are more resilient and better able to absorb strength from their general training. After 30, the body's affinity for fitness begins to wean and bone density slowly becomes more and more important.

Gender plays a role, too. Generally speaking, men genetically maintain strength above that of their female counterparts. That said, resistance training may provide more value for women than men when it comes to TRI.

Prior strength training is another variable that must be considered. If your background is in the weight room and you have significant strength and muscle mass, your time may be better spent in TRI specific/flexibility conditioning. If you are very lean and your muscles begin to fatigue quickly during aerobic training, you may really benefit from pumping some iron.

Coaches' Corner

Many triathletes fear that their body will bulk up if they lift weights. Really, it's not likely that you'll gain much weight. The TRI strategy of resistance training is on the opposite end of the spectrum from a body builder's type of program. If you happen to put on a few pounds, the performance benefits will definitely be worth it!.

If your schedule only has time for X hours and you're faced with a choice between giving up a TRI workout or a weight lifting workout, sacrifice the gym time. In a perfect world, no workout would be sacrificed and every workout would receive the same focus and attention.

Many variables—all very specific and individual to you—will impact your lifting schedule and goals. However, generally speaking, we believe that augmenting TRI with resistance training is the greatest path to peak performance.

How Do I Do It?

How should you weight train? In addition to the aforementioned guidelines, your training should …

♦ Start gradually—ease into your training.

♦ Be controlled—always have control of the load.

♦ Utilize a full range of motion—this provides optimal gains.

♦ Incorporate variety—mix up the order, change loads, change angles (but always keep it safe!).

> **Training Tips**
>
> Whenever possible, mimic specific TRI movements during weight training exercises. For example, if you were doing pull-ups, position your hands where they would be during swimming. Or if you're performing squats or leg press, have your feet about the same width as your bike pedals. This helps condition your body at specific angles most conducive to TRI.

Something else to consider is core conditioning. The core refers to your body's center—your abdominal and lower back muscles—and comes into play in all three TRI disciplines. A strong core generates power in the swim, helps hold your position on the bike, and aids in posture during the run. We strongly believe you should include core activities whenever possible.

Workouts

We have included several suggested exercises in the following sections. *Prior to attempting any of these programs, first get approval from your doctor. Then, perform all the exercises with proper technique.* If any exercise causes you joint pain, *stop immediately* and move to the next one.

We've included 14 total movements (one circuit). Generally speaking, we recommend you perform 8 to 12 reps of each exercise, for 1 or 2 sets, 2 or 3 times a week. If you want to complete two sets, you could either complete a full circuit with one set each exercise and then repeat, or you could do two sets of each movement before going to the next. We prefer completing a full circuit.

> **Gravel Ahead**
>
> Listen to your body as you work out, especially in the beginning. It knows how far it can go—and when you've pushed too far. *This is hard* is an okay thought to have while working out; *This really hurts* is not.

In general, we have alternated upper body movements with lower body ones. This is an ideal way to maximize and balance endurance with recovery. It helps maintain intensity while giving specific regions rest while you work others; providing you with an efficient workout session. And one other thing worth mentioning, you should not lift weights (same muscle groups) two days in a row as your muscles need time to recover and rebuild.

Here's the circuit, in order: squat, lat pull-down, leg extension, bench press, leg curl, dip, lunge, cable row, seated calf raise, push down, dumbbell curl, ball crunch, lateral raise, and back extension.

Each exercise is broken out into a *preparation* and a *movement* section. The preparation material deals with general setup while the movement text outlines the specific exercise in detail. If we mention "activating" a muscle/body part, that simply means you'll be flexing or tightening that area. Remember, a good rule of thumb is 8 to 12 reps per set (or whatever you feel comfortable with)—let's get pumped! Following your warm-up …

Squat

Preparation: Position yourself under the bar, resting it on your upper back muscles. Grab the bar with your hands just outside of shoulder width. Lift the weight off the rack, and take a step back to your starting position where your feet are planted about shoulder-width apart, pointing straight ahead, and knees over your second and third toes. Your head should be in line with your spine.

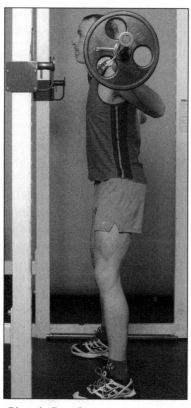 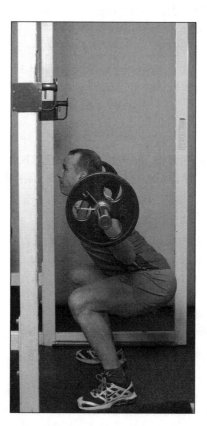

(Photos by Peter Baiamonte)

Movement: Activate your core and glutes while you begin the descent by bending at the knees/hips. Maintain about a 45-degree angle (from vertical) with your trunk. Squat as deep as you can with comfort and without compromising form. Then press up through your heels, maintaining proper body alignment. When you reach the top, keep a slight knee bend.

Lat Pull-Down

Preparation: Grab the bar (overhand grip) just outside of shoulder-width. Sit on the seat, and secure your legs under the knee pads.

Movement: Maintain a slight backward trunk lean as you pull the bar down to your chest (collarbone area). Pause briefly as you squeeze your shoulder blades together. Avoid creating momentum by swinging and jerking; always stay in control of the weight.

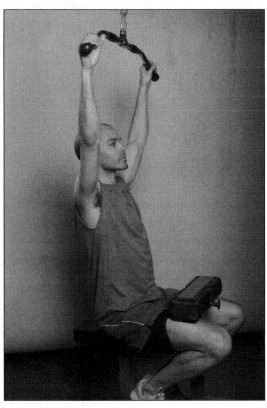
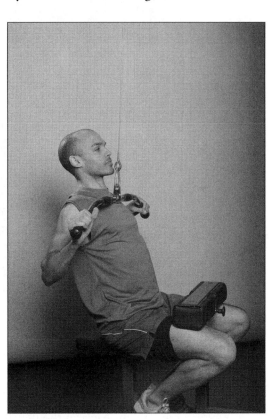

(Photos by Peter Baiamonte)

Leg Extension

Preparation: Sit in the seat with your back flat against the vertical pad and your shins up against the leg pads just above your ankles. In the start position, your hips, knees, and ankles should form a 90-degree angle.

Movement: Extend your lower legs until they're nearly straight. Squeeze the thigh muscles, pause there, and then lower the load while under control. Keep your butt and back in their original placements. Avoid lifting your hips during the movement.

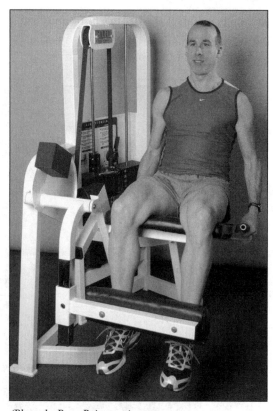 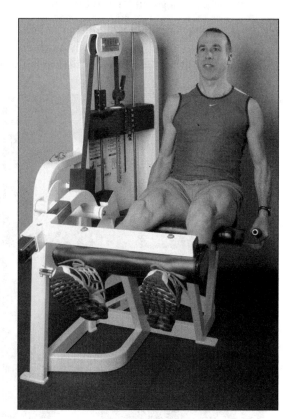

(Photos by Peter Baiamonte)

Bench Press

Preparation: Lie on your back on the bench. Position yourself to where you'll have room to lift the weight without hitting the upright bar rests. Place your feet flat on the floor or balance them on the bench as shown. Grab the bar just outside of shoulder-width apart.

Movement: Lift the bar off the uprights and hold it over your chest. Lower it to your chest, pause, and return it to the starting position. Always maintain control of the weight. Do not bounce it off your chest, and remember to breathe throughout the movement.

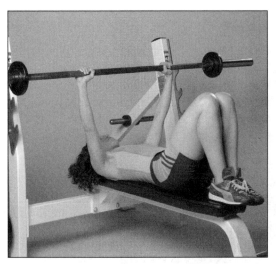
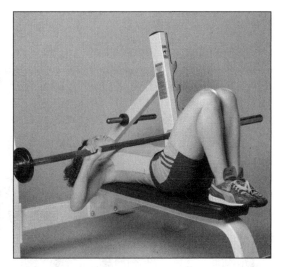

(Photos by Peter Baiamonte)

Leg Curl

Preparation: Lie face down on the machine, and place your lower legs up against the leg pads just above your heels. Your knees should be off of the pad rest. Grab the handles for support. Your head should be either down with your chin/forehead resting on the pad or lifted slightly off the pad.

Movement: Bend your legs at your knees lifting the weight as high as you can. Pause and then slowly return to the starting position. Keep your pelvis and thighs in constant contact with the pad throughout the movement. Also, maintain your chosen head alignment during the move.

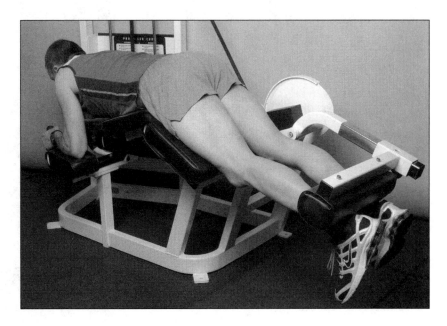

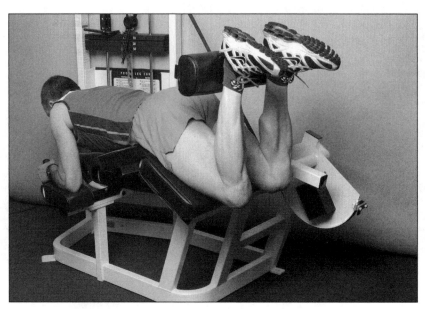

(Photos by Peter Baiamonte)

Dip

Preparation: Hoist yourself onto the parallel bars/handles. Allow your body to drop to where you are perpendicular to the floor. Bend your knees and cross your ankles for comfort.

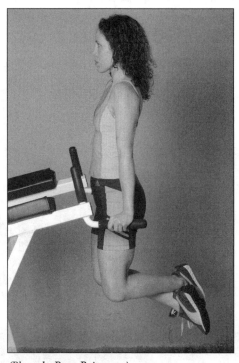 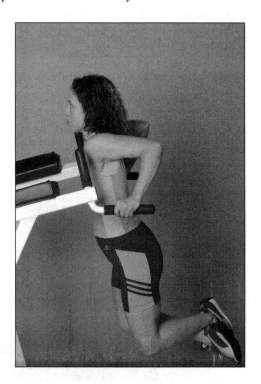

(Photos by Peter Baiamonte)

Movement: Slowly lower yourself as deep as you can; ideally, until your upper arms are parallel to the floor. Push back until your elbows are almost straight but not locked. Maintaining a more vertical body alignment primarily works your triceps. If you lean forward and flare your elbows out, you'll recruit chest and shoulder muscles.

Lunge

Preparation: It's optional to use dumbbells for added resistance. If so, hold two dumbbells at your side with palms facing in. Stand with your feet just inside of shoulder-width.

Movement: Make a stride with your right leg. Then bend at the knees until your right leg forms a 90-degree angle. Be sure not to extend your knee past your toes. Return to the starting position and switch legs. Maintain an upright torso throughout the movement.

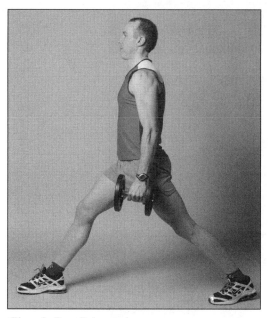 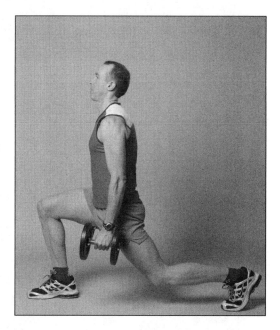

(Photos by Peter Baiamonte)

Cable Row

Preparation: Sit down and position your feet on the platform. Grab the handle with extended arms. Your knees are slightly bent.

Movement: Pull the handle to your midsection. Pause and squeeze your shoulder blades together. Slowly return to the starting position. Keep your back erect and your abdominals tight.

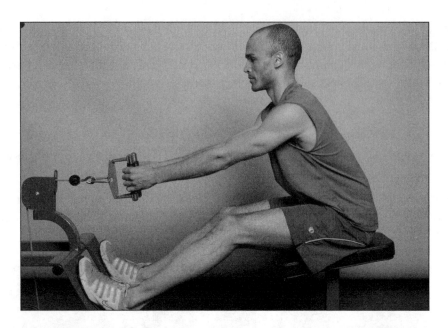

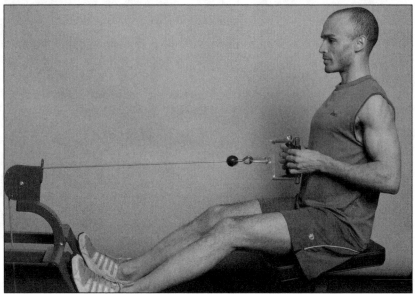

(Photos by Peter Baiamonte)

Seated Calf Raise

Preparation: Sit with your back erect, your knees under the pads, and balls of your feet on the edge of the foot plate. Grab onto the handles only for comfort and balance. Do not cheat during the movement by pulling on them.

Movement: Release the support and lower your heels as far as you can. Then lift your heels as far as you can and without pausing, lower back to the starting position.

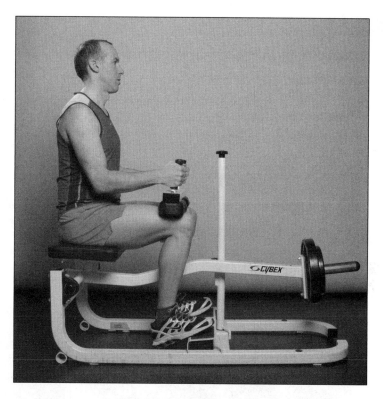

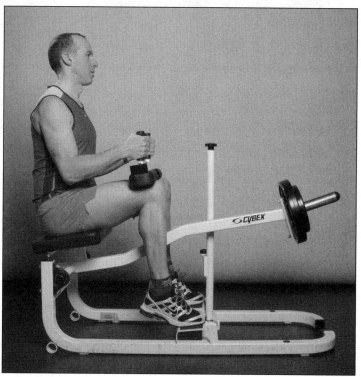

(Photos by Peter Baiamonte)

Pushdown

Preparation: Stand erect in front of the machine and grab the handle. Keep your elbows close to your sides. They should also be near to a 90-degree angle.

Movement: Straighten your arms. Pause and be sure to get a good squeeze at the bottom. Then slowly return to the starting position. Keep your upper arms and torso in a fixed position during this movement.

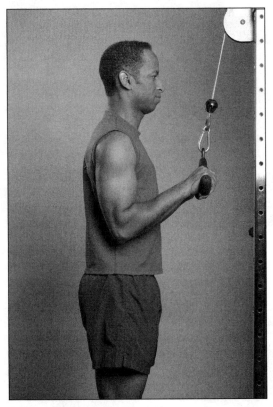 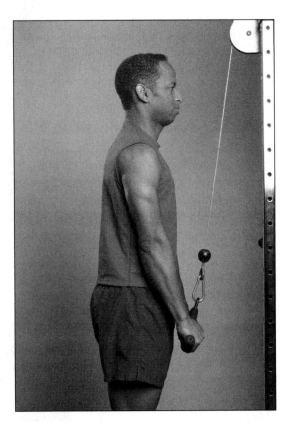

(Photos by Peter Baiamonte)

Dumbbell Curl

Preparation: Sit tall with a dumbbell in each hand (facing inward). Activate your abdominals and keep your elbows close to your sides.

Movement: Begin to bend your elbows while rotating your wrists so your palms are facing upward. Raise the weights as high as you can without allowing forward motion by your elbows. Pause, squeeze, and with control return to the starting position as you rotate your wrists/ palms back to the inward position.

Tip: Completely straighten your arms by flexing your triceps at the end of each rep, ensuring you are working your bicep in a full range of motion.

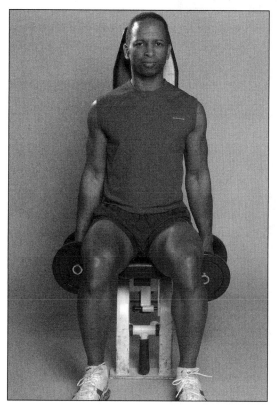 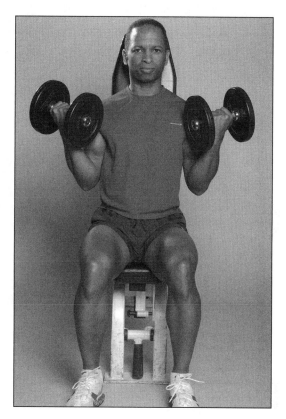

(Photos by Peter Baiamonte)

Ball Crunch

Preparation: Lie on your back on the Swiss (a.k.a. Stability) ball with your fingers behind your ears. Place your feet flat on the floor about hip-width apart.

Movement: Contract your abdominals and raise your head and shoulders. Crunch your rib cage toward your pelvis. Pause, and slowly return to the starting position. Activate your abs during both the lifting and lowering phases.

Tip: Exhale forcefully at the top of the movement, which gives your abs a little extra work. This exercise can exceed the rep range of 8-12. Feel free to crunch until you feel the burn.

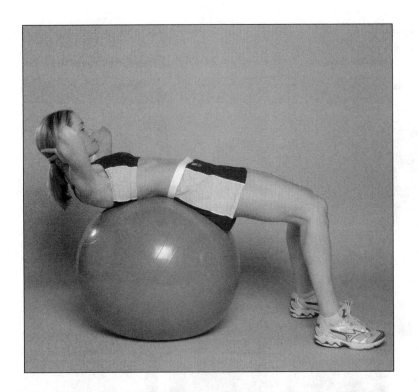

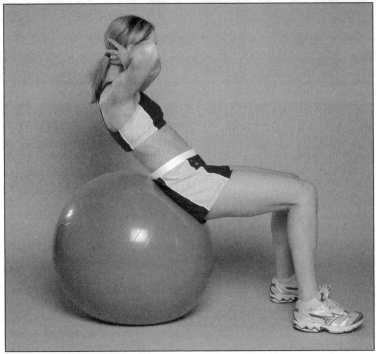

(Photos by Peter Baiamonte)

Lateral Raise

Preparation: Sit on the end of a bench holding two dumbbells at your sides (palms facing inward). Place your feet flat on the floor for stability. Your torso is erect. Keep a slight bend to your elbows.

Movement: Raise the dumbbells out to your sides until the upper arms are parallel to the floor. Pause, and slowly return to the starting position.

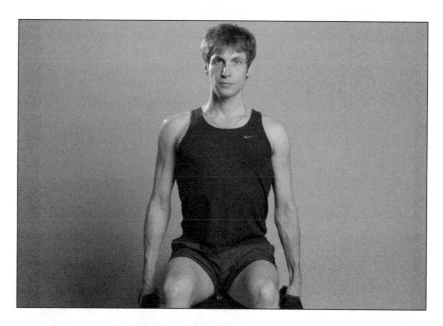

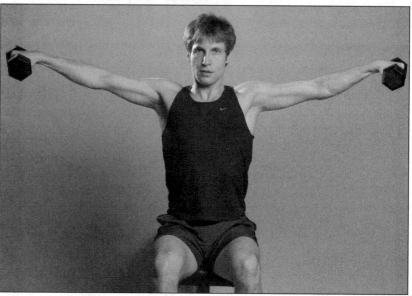

(Photos by Peter Baiamonte)

Back Extension

Preparation: Secure your feet on the platform or under the leg anchors, depending on the equipment. Bend at the waist and let your torso hang. Keep your head in alignment with your spine. Cross your arms in front. As an option, you can increase the difficulty by holding your hands behind your head or holding a medicine ball to your chest.

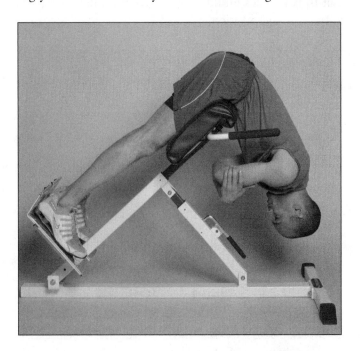

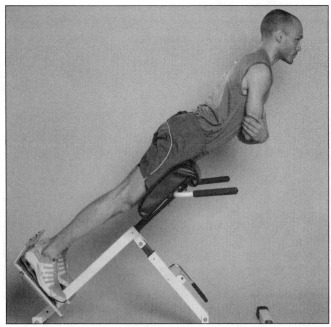

(Photos by Peter Baiamonte)

Movement: Raise your torso up until it is straight with the rest of your body. Pause, and slowly return to the starting position. Do not bounce or swing. Always stay in control of your weight.

Tip: Similar to Ball Crunch, adjust the reps as necessary.

Stretch It Out

You've probably heard that you should stretch when exercising, but sometimes that seems like an extra step in your already-full life. Try to find the time! Stretching helps you achieving your personal best while helping prevent injuries. Consider stretching a cardinal contributing factor in your overall peak performance pursuit.

Why Stretch?

Stretching makes you flexible, and good *flexibility* has been linked with everything from increased performance, to reduced chance of injury, to better recovery, to improved muscular balance and postural awareness. Stretching works! When you apply force at the right intensities, in appropriate durations, and with some frequency, you increase connective tissue flexibility. Being more flexible is directly related to being a better TRI version of yourself.

def•i•ni•tion

Flexibility is the range of motion within a joint. It comes from the Latin *flexibilis,* which means "to bend."

When Do I Stretch?

The best time to stretch is when your muscles are warm, such as right after your workout session. Studies suggest that performing the same stretching steps when your body's tissue temperature is slightly elevated versus normal produces a greater permanent (plastic) deformation. That's the goal. Performing the same steps with a cooler tissue temperature only produces temporary tissue elongation. Therefore, after a workout session, cool down and flow right into your stretching routine while your body temperature is still elevated and your muscles are supple. You can't bend steel without heating it first!

As with resistance training, many schools of thought exist when it comes to stretching. Some believe you should only have a focused session two to three times a week. Others believe you should stretch every day. Listen to your body and find out what works best for you. Spending a few minutes stretching things out can save you hours and even days in recovery or injury.

Coaches' Corner

To put some fun in your stretching routine, try a yoga or Pilates class. Taking a couple classes a week is a great way to augment your brief postworkout stretch sessions.

You could also opt to designate a day or two every week to spend more time stretching. Perhaps this is when you add more sets and duration to each stretch. For example, if you perform 1 set at 30 seconds' duration of each stretch postworkout, you could add 2 or 3 more sets at 60 seconds duration on these designated days. If you're going to stretch at a time not directly following a workout, perform a 5- to 10-minute warm-up.

How Do I Stretch?

Three popular types of stretching techniques are: static, dynamic, and proprioceptive neuro-muscular facilitation (PNF)

Static stretching is the preferred and most widely accepted method of stretching. It involves a slow, gradual, low-intensity stretch. The intensity is the point at which you begin to feel a slight discomfort—*not* pain. Generally, you would hold a stretch for 10 to 30 seconds and repeat each stretch 2 to 4 times.

Dynamic stretching is an active stretch done through a full range of motion. It is done in a slow and controlled manner. The theory behind it is to mimic activities that are dynamic in nature such as a golf swing.

PNF is composed of many strategies. One of the more commonly used aspects of it deals with a contract-relax sequence. Essentially, you would flex (contract) with maximum force or resistance at the end point of a limb's range of motion. This is an isometric movement. You would hold it for approximately 5 to 10 seconds and then relax and apply an easy stretch. You can perform this sequence of contracting and relaxing several times, and it's best performed with a partner. PNF is a more complicated method, and therefore, it's important to do your due diligence before attempting it. If you're interested in PNF, we suggest doing further research before you incorporate it into your TRI program.

Training Tips _____

Degree of flexibility decreases with age. As people get older, there's a shift in colla-gen fibers and in overall hydration in and around soft tissue structures. If you're under 30, you probably won't need to hold your stretches as long as someone who is over 30. After the age of 30, you need to start increasing the time you hold your stretches (up to 60 seconds) to receive the same benefits.

When stretching, it's important to remember the following tenants:

- Low-intensity, long-duration stretching is most conducive for lasting benefits.

- Warming your tissue temperature prior to stretching contributes to increased range of motion and lasting benefits.

- Target specific joints and muscle groups when you stretch, and maintain that specific focus.

- Hold most stretches for a minimum of 10 seconds and up to 60 seconds; repeat each 2 to 4 times.

◆ Give tighter areas extra attention, spending more duration or frequency there.

◆ Breathe slowly and deeply through the stretches, maintaining an even ratio of inhalations to exhalations.

Flexibility is an integral part of your overall fitness equation. Given the movements of swim, bike, and run, stretching is especially important for those training for TRI. Flexible knees and hips better extend during your cycling stroke. Pliable shoulders help you in swimming. Supple hamstrings aid on the bike. Flexible quadriceps facilitate running efficiency. Static or slow steady stretching at low intensity is the most favorable technique you can employ. Engaging in a regular stretching program reaps many benefits such as increased performance, decreased recovery time, and reduced risk of injury. Always, always make time for stretching.

Movements

In the following sections, we go over some good stretches that hit the major muscle groups.

Quadriceps

1. Stand up, holding onto something for balance with one hand if necessary.

2. With your free hand, grasp your corresponding upper foot/ankle, and bring your heel toward your butt. Keep your knees adjacent to one another.

3. Maintain alignment as you pull back, stretching your quad muscle.

4. Hold for 30 to 60 seconds and then switch legs.

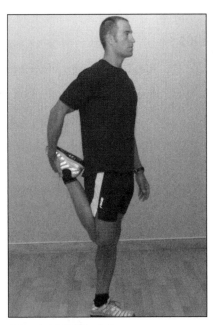

(Photo by Todd Schoelen)

Hamstrings

1. Lie on your back, with one leg down and the other held up using a towel wrapped around your foot.

2. Keep your down leg grounded flat on the floor as you bring your other one up and back.

3. Press the heel of your raised leg up toward the ceiling and feel the stretch in the back of your leg.

4. Hold for 30 to 60 seconds and then switch legs.

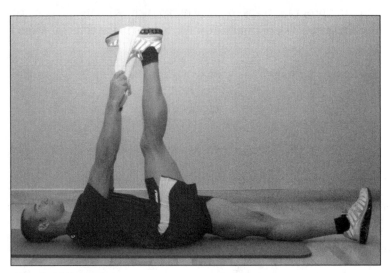

(Photo by Todd Schoelen)

Calves

1. Stand up, using a chair or wall for support.

2. Place the toes of one foot up against a wall or other object, keeping your heel down.

3. Use your back leg/foot for balance and support.

4. Stand erect and lean in toward the wall until you feel tension in the calf of your front foot.

5. Hold for 30 to 60 seconds and then switch legs.

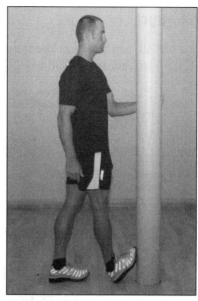

(Photo by Todd Schoelen)

Pure Hip

1. Lie on your back, perpendicular to a wall, your left leg bent at 90 degrees, and your left foot flat against the wall.

2. Place your right ankle just below your left knee with your right hand resting on your right knee (like you're in a chair, crossing your legs).

3. Press your right hand into your right knee and toward the wall.

4. Use your left hand for balance or support on the floor or on your left leg or hip. You should feel the stretch in your right hip.

5. Hold for 30 to 60 seconds and then switch sides.

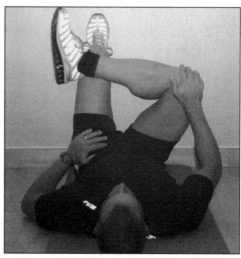

(Photo by Todd Schoelen)

Hip Flexors

1. Place a towel on the floor and drop a knee down to it as you perform a lunge. Your other knee should be directly over your foot and ankle, not beyond.

2. Place your hands on your thigh for support.

3. Drop your hips and feel the stretch.

4. Hold for 30 to 60 seconds and then switch legs.

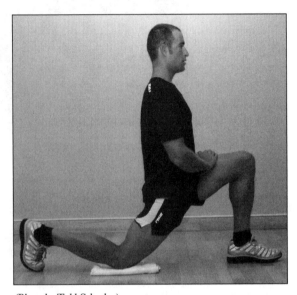

(Photo by Todd Schoelen)

Sitting Spinal Twist (a.k.a. Pretzel)

1. Sit tall on the floor with both legs out in front of you.

2. Pick up your right leg, bending it, and drop your right foot down on the outside of your left knee.

3. Place your right hand on the floor behind your right buttock for support.

4. While twisting to your right, bring your left arm across your right knee and rest your left hand on your left leg, and gaze out over your right shoulder.

5. Apply passive or gentle pressure between your left upper arm and right knee.

6. Hold for 30 to 60 seconds and then switch sides.

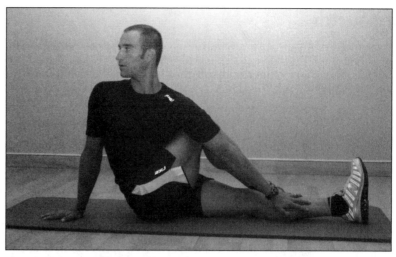

(Photo by Todd Schoelen)

Lower Back (aka Cat Stretch)

1. Begin in an all-fours position.

2. Position your hands under your shoulders about shoulder width apart and your knees under your hips about hip width apart.

3. Keep a slight bend in your elbows with your fingers facing forward.

4. Gently round your back. Feel the stretch throughout your spine as you lengthen your shoulders and back.

5. Hold for 30 to 60 seconds.

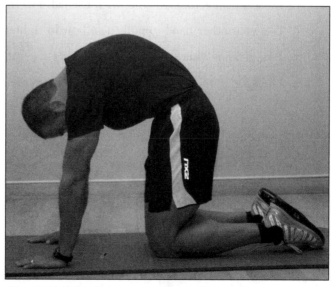

(Photo by Todd Schoelen)

Torso Stretch

1. Lie on your stomach and place your hands and arms as if you were doing a push-up.

2. Raise your upper body off the floor while keeping your hips and lower body in contact with the floor. Feel the stretch open up your core.

3. Hold for 30 to 60 seconds.

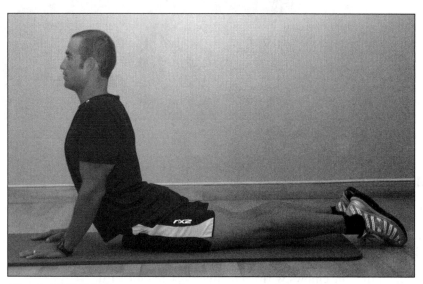

(Photo by Todd Schoelen)

Triceps Stretch

1. Raise a bent arm, elbow up, with the palm of that hand resting on your back.

2. Use your other hand to pull the elbow in tighter.

3. Find a point where you feel it stretching the back of the upper arm.

4. Hold for 30 to 60 seconds and then switch arms.

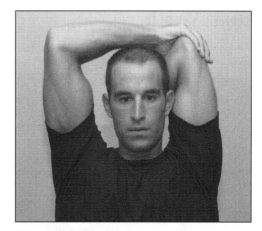

(Photo by Todd Schoelen)

Shoulder Opener

1. Stand sideways next to a wall with your left hand resting on the wall, your fingertips pointing upward or slightly backward about shoulder height.

2. Hold that arm position and then slowly twist your upper body away from the wall.

3. Hold for 30 to 60 seconds and then switch sides.

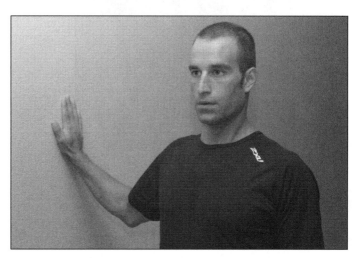

(Photo by Todd Schoelen)

Posterior Shoulder

1. Relax your shoulders and let them drop down.

2. Bring your left arm across your chest, parallel to the floor.

3. Use your right arm to help apply gentle pressure toward your body.

4. Hold for 30 to 60 seconds and then switch arms.

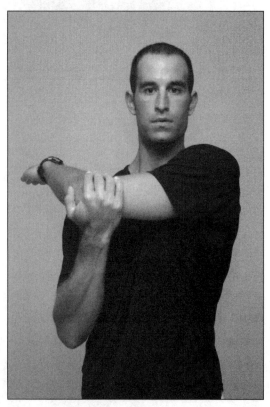

(Photo by Todd Schoelen)

Neck

1. Stand or sit erect, and wrap one arm over the top of your head.

2. Place the hand of the raised arm on your head and apply passive pressure. Feel the stretch in the side of your neck.

3. Hold for 30 to 60 seconds and then switch sides.

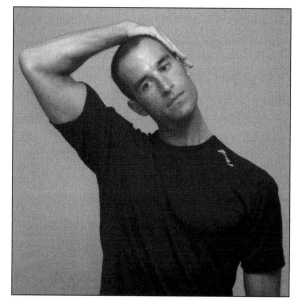

(Photo by Todd Schoelen)

Resistance and flexibility training are, in most cases, ideal ways to augment TRI conditioning. They challenge your body in ways that the three sports of TRI alone cannot. The results and benefits are many—and not just in the short-term. These principles can help improve your physical quality of life from now onward. Balancing resistance training, flexibility, and TRI-specific conditioning is the best way to reaching your full active lifestyle potential.

The Least You Need to Know

◆ Resistance training has been shown to improve strength, bone density, overall TRI peak performance and is also linked to the reduced chance of injury.

◆ Always progress gradually, maintain control of the load, and perform movements in a full range of motion.

◆ Flexibility conditioning has been connected with everything from increased performance, to reduced chance of injury, to better recovery, to improved muscular balance and postural awareness.

◆ Low-intensity, long-duration stretching is most conducive for lasting benefits.

◆ Stretch after a warm-up or workout when your body's tissue temperatures are above normal.

Chapter 11

Minding Your R&R

In This Chapter

- ◆ Understanding the mind-body connection
- ◆ Learning the aspects of mental conditioning and improving self-belief
- ◆ Why rest and recovery are sometimes overlooked
- ◆ Building R&R into your TRI training

The body follows where the mind leads. So much attention is paid to the physical side of sports, but very little is given to the mental component. It's critical, though, to mentally prepare yourself for the challenge of triathlon. Your mind-set plays a major role in both training and racing, especially as intensity and distance increase.

Just as important as understanding the mind game is knowing "when to say when." If you push yourself too hard, you risk overtraining, burnout, illness, and injury. Throughout your triathlon season, you'll need to incorporate both planned and unplanned breaks into your schedule. After putting in long or intense training, your body needs some time to build itself back up and absorb all the benefits of those workouts. You'll need to become comfortable with this concept: sometimes less is more.

In this chapter, we first take a look at "going mental" and then finish up with some information on working in some good R&R.

The Mind Game

At first glance, TRI appears to be a purely physical sport—you swim, bike, and run. Oh … and you sometimes change clothes in between. But when you peel back a couple layers, you quickly realize that so much more is involved in TRI than you might have first noticed.

TRI isn't just your physical body going through the motions; your powerful psyche directs each step of the way. Your mind is like a conductor leading a symphony; without this guidance and direction, there would just be sound. With coordination, however, there's a blend of harmony and balance.

def•i•ni•tion

Psychosomatic is anything involving a mind and body connection.

The best way to tap into the power of your mind is by first making the connection between mind and body. When you become cognizant of the *psychosomatic* link, you can leverage it. The mind can be an ally or an adversary, depending on how you learn to work with it. When you unite your physical and mental forces, there's nothing you can't do.

Some of the talent on your mental team includes attitude, motivation, focus, and determination. These factors work together to create a solid mental state. Let's meet each of them.

Attitude: They Say It's Everything

You've probably heard the clichés:

> Attitude is everything.

> Life is 10 percent what happens to you and 90 percent how you deal with what happens.

Cliché or not, there's a lot of truth in these statements. Life *is* full of challenges; we're defined by how we choose to deal with the obstacles that stand in our way.

The same goes for TRI. You'll experience all three types of TRI days: the good, the bad, and the ugly. Having the right attitude throughout makes the difference between just going through the motions and finishing with a TRI-umphant smile.

What's My Motivation?

Maintaining high levels of motivation is a crucial step in your TRI experience—it can make the difference between waking up for an early workout and hitting the snooze button for the third time. At times throughout your training, your motivation will be tested. It's in these moments when you need a mental boost. Pull out your TRI goal/training program. Remind yourself that you have a plan and a purpose for all your hard work.

Here are some other motivational strategies to keep you moving along:

◆ Build milestones into your overall goal, such as losing *X* percent of body fat.

◆ Find a workout partner who helps hold you accountable.

◆ When appropriate and safe, work out to your favorite music.

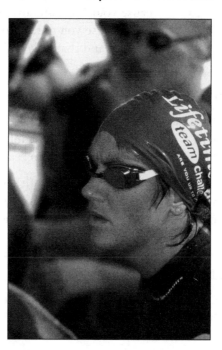

Olympic triathlete Barb Lindquist finds her mental zone before a race.

(Photo by Lois Schwartz)

Coaches' Corner

A personal mantra can help you move forward during difficult workouts. You don't need to speak the mantra out loud, but having a simple phrase that triggers added motivation when things get rough can be a real lifesaver. Some people repeat the refrain of a favorite song; some repeat a single word on a rhythm (*de-ter-mi-na-tion, de-ter-mi-na-tion*); others use an inspirational phrase. When the going gets tough for Colin, he remembers the TV broadcast of the beginning of a football game that showed an entire team united as one, focused, jumping up and down, and chanting his mantra: "Got to go to work ... got to go to work ..." Repeating that phrase helps Colin refocus and stay on course when things get rough.

Focus ... Focus ...

The ability to focus is another integral mental component. When the going gets tough, the tough get focused. Instead of letting your mind wander into a negative abyss, concentrate on what's happening in the here and now. If you're facing a killer headwind on the bike ... and you're tired ... and the temperature is off the charts, *do not despair*. Get focused! Think about your pedal stroke. Are you concentrating on pressing force down through the pedal and

def•i•ni•tion

Economy is the efficiency in which you perform an activity. In TRI, you swim, bike, and run. Your economy is how efficiently your body works to get you from point A to point B.

circulating around in little circles? Are you wasting any energy in your shoulders or hands? Can you get more aerodynamic by dropping down into your aerobars?

It's pointless to feel depressed and helpless about how tough you have it. Taking your focus away from the race could cause your form and overall *economy* to suffer. That, in turn, could cause you to take longer to finish off the difficult stretch, and that only compounds the issue.

Maintain Your Determination

Determination tops off our winning mental formula. What is your level of commitment to the goal? Is it in harmony with your lifestyle and schedule? What does accomplishing this goal mean to you? What are you willing to give up to reach it?

Perhaps TRI serves as a hobby; something you do with your friends. Maybe it's a lifestyle you've chosen to maintain overall fitness. Whatever drives you to the sport, determination keeps you giving 110 percent when part of you would rather kick back on the couch and watch TV.

Gravel Ahead

It's important for you to fully commit to your goals. If you're only partially dedicated, your subconscious will veto the less-than-true commitment and you might eventually find yourself derailed from achieving your goal.

Picture Yourself Succeeding

Don't just think you can; *know* you can. Believe in yourself. Have confidence in your abilities to achieve your goals and dreams. The magic behind all great accomplishments begins with this self-belief. Sometimes we feel down on ourselves and doubt our abilities, but that's normal. When it happens, take a step back and regroup by replacing the negative thoughts with positive ones and remember you can accomplish anything with the right state of mind.

A lot of research supports the power of visualization. The general theory is that thought has the ability to create feelings and emotions that impact behavior and, ultimately, reality. In other words, when you think about success day in and day out, you eventually will create that success.

Training Tips

If you fill your head with negative thoughts, you'll eventually make those negative thoughts your reality. Think positive. *Know* you can do this!

It all begins with a single thought. If you wake up every morning, look yourself in the mirror, and say, "I'm going to …" Eventually it will happen. The power of thought and intention is very real and can very easily be applied to TRI. Visualize yourself in the swim: your stroke is smooth, your breathing is under control, and you found a good draft off someone's feet. Imagine having a great T1, bike segment, T2, and run. Imagine crossing the finish line. Put those strong positive beliefs out there. When you do, the door to manifesting these beliefs in reality opens to you.

Focus on What's in Your Control

Much of the anxiety and doubt that creeps into our heads is wasted energy. If you stop and think about these negative thoughts, you'll find many of them fall into the "outside your control" category. If it's not in your control, you're wasting precious time and energy worrying about it. Once you've dubbed it futile, shift your attention on what you *can* control. Nothing else matters. For example, if you're in a race and the start of your age group wave is delayed, don't panic or stress out. There's nothing you can do about starting on schedule. Take advantage of the extra time to meditate, stay hydrated, listen to your MP3 player, talk with a TRI neighbor, etc.

Here's a breakdown of each category—what's in your control and what you're better off not worrying about.

Out of Your Control	In Your Control
Weather	Mental state
Race course (aid stations, markings and signage, volunteers)	Pacing
Swim conditions (swells, currents, competitors)	Nutrition/hydration
Bike conditions (wind, potholes, debris, flat tires, competitors)	Equipment (in working order)
Run conditions (surfaces, topography, competitors)	Technique
	Clothing
	Proper sunscreen and lube application
	Race strategy and knowledge of the course

When you have a clear understanding of the difference between what is in your control and what's out of your control, you'll be prepared to maximize your mental facilities. Label it, sort it into the right category, and deal with it appropriately.

Face Your Fear

To make the best of your TRI experience, learn to deal with any lingering fears you might have. Only after you identify your fears and deal with them are you able to evolve in TRI and in life. Fears show up differently for everyone. Some fear open-water swims, fast descents on the bike, or more generally, their overall race results. It's up to you to face the things you fear and learn how to process them. You need to accept that fear, act on it, or put it in perspective.

Accept the fact that you're nervous or scared. Most triathletes, if they're honest, admit to being nervous about some aspect in TRI training or racing. Nervousness is natural, and as long as you learn to control and channel this emotion, it can't hurt you.

If your fear is more intense and focused, you'll need to face it head-on (act). If swimming in open water makes you hyperventilate with terror, you'll need to get past it if you want to be a triathlete (unless you can find some shorter indoor TRIs to take part in). Otherwise, you might find yourself in a panic during a race. The best way to get over such a fear is by swimming the open water over and over again. Go for a swim with someone who can help you through this challenge. Wear a wetsuit and only go out a short distance. Do this until you're confident. Being comfortable in everything you do is critical in your overall TRI success.

> **Coaches' Corner**
>
> Almost all fear is rooted in the lack of trust in ourselves. When you learn to believe in yourself, you'll find the confidence to overcome fear.

> **Training Tips**
>
> There's nothing wrong with talking to yourself. Sometimes when things get tough out on a training session or race, you'll feel the need to talk to yourself. That's totally normal. If you start to lose focus and ramble however, it might be a good time to end your monologue and concentrate on your mantra.

Gaining perspective on a situation can also play a key role. Ask yourself what you're afraid of and why. Then apply a sense of reality to it. If you're scared of not meeting your own race expectations, try to put that fear into context. If you don't finish in the time you wanted (we advocate not having a time goal) or feeling the way you wanted, you'll have a tremendous learning opportunity. You might learn something about your training strategy and how you can adjust it the next time around. As long as you document any lessons learned and utilize them next time around, almost all race experiences can help you.

Putting perspective around the fear should help you control it. In the grand scheme of things, is this fear worthy of your time and stress? Is it a big deal? Perhaps, once you take a step back, you'll realize the fear is superficial and you can get past it. Your head is the source of creating your reality. Always stay optimistic. Believe.

The Psychological Perspective

When you get into training and racing, it becomes very natural to get sucked into the vortex of more, more, more—more miles, more yards, more intensity …. It's important to understand how the mind and the ego can work against you if you're not careful. You could easily fall into a routine of consistent workouts. Your body will get stronger, you might shed some pounds, and you might feel the "TRI high" from endorphins popping. Whatever the case, it's easy to slip into this addictive mentality. Triathletes can get to the point where if they're not working out once or twice a day, they feel awkward and unnatural. Some might think, *What do you mean take the day off? I'll get weak, gain weight, and have poor performance in my next race.*

This is a very real phenomenon and is not always easily understood. When it's happening to you, you might be too close to see it objectively. When you see it happen to someone else (especially if you're not as active), it's hard to comprehend. Knowing about this tendency up front might help keep you on the right track with smart and safe training practices.

Give Yourself Time Off

One of the ways to be sure you're getting enough rest and recovery is to schedule it in your training plan. Building recovery into your schedule is critical. Many triathletes neglect sufficient amounts of recovery unless they're being monitored by a coach. Even then, we've seen cases where individuals sneak in workouts when they should be riding the couch, regardless of advice. This is a mind-set that needs to be changed—now. The right amount of rest is your friend.

Rest Days

One way to work recovery into your schedule is by designating a certain day(s) off per week. At a minimum, have at least one day off. You can move or adjust the day(s) based on your other responsibilities (career, family, social, travel, other); or you can have a fixed day (every Friday is a rest day). It depends on you and your life and the signals you get from your body.

When you're just starting your training, it might be difficult to make yourself rest ... especially if you have some extra time where a workout would fit perfectly. Try to use the time to hang out with your family, call a friend, read a novel, or catch up on the news. (We'll schedule specific rest days into your training plan, but don't be afraid to move them around if necessary.)

> **Coaches' Corner**
>
> If you absolutely must work out on a designated rest day, a nice, easy swim is your best bet. As long as you keep the intensity low, an easy swim makes the least impact on your body.

Active Recovery Workouts

Active recovery workouts are a critical component of the recovery process. We spread these into your schedule, usually on a day following a training session that places a large demand on your body (time or intensity).

Although an active recovery session might seem too slow or almost effortless (easy bike or easy swim with a focus on technique), the sessions cause

def•i•ni•tion

> An **active recovery workout** is a low-intensity session, such as an easy bike or swim with more of a focus on technique. It can speed up recovery by flushing fatigued areas with blood and nutrients.

blood flow to increase to the traumatized muscles. Nutrients and hormones are carried in the blood and contribute to overall recovery.

Recovery Weeks

Beyond specific rest days and active recovery workouts, we also build recovery weeks into your schedule, usually every fourth week or so. During a recovery week, you drop down the volume and intensity a bit and give your body a more extended period to regenerate.

If a rest day is hard for a triathlete to swallow, a recovery week might present even more of a challenge. The week will seem too easy, and you might become worried that you're not doing enough training. Don't panic! Your body will use this time to get ready for the challenges that lay ahead. Hopefully, when a recovery week comes up in the schedule, your body will let you know it's ready for some rest.

Training Tips _____

To help with muscle recovery, triathletes of all fitness levels can benefit from getting a massage on a regular basis. Prices vary, but if you find a student masseuse who needs more hands-on hours as part of his or her training, you can get some great rates.

Catch Some ZZZs!

Although often overlooked, sleep is a critical element in your training. Your body uses the time you're out to rejuvenate itself. When training volume increases, so should sleep. If you were a 7-hour-a-night sleeper before training, you might now require 8.

The best way to catch more ZZZs is to incorporate gradual changes into your schedule. You might try going to bed 30 minutes earlier than normal at night. You could try to add sleep to your day by taking a power nap at lunch. If it works into your day, go for it. Sleep long enough to feel refreshed, but not so long that you won't be able to sleep at night. This extra sleep will do wonders for recovery and your overall energy levels. Enjoy!

Can't nap during the day, you say? Have trouble going to bed early? Here are some tips for falling asleep:

♦ Get to bed at or near the same time each night.

♦ Avoid working out too close to bedtime ("too close" varies for different people; 2 hours is a safe bet for many ... but some can workout and then go straight to sleep).

♦ Try reading just before bedtime to relax your mind.

♦ Take a warm bath.

♦ Make the room conducive: dark, cool, and comfortable.

♦ Drink a cup of herbal tea or warm milk as you near bedtime.

Coaches' Corner
Similar to caloric intake, the more you train, the more sleep you need to meet the demands placed on your body.

Some people turn to pharmaceutical companies when sleep is elusive. If you've been taking some sort of sleep aid before you begin training with a doctor's recommendation, you can, of course, continue to do so. However, many people who have trouble sleeping find that sleep comes easier when exercise is added to their weekly routine. Pushing the body physically during the day makes it more susceptible to the sandman at night. If you do utilize any sort of sleeping aid, just be aware that it may be more difficult for you to get your body cranked up for any early morning workouts. Also, be careful. There's been a lot of chatter lately about the addictive quality of these aids.

Know When to Say When

Some recovery days and weeks are specifically scheduled in your TRI training, but that schedule is not the end-all, be-all. Listen to your body. What signals is it sending you? How do you really feel? This can be a very difficult thing to master and comply with. Remember, the ego and psyche may be working against you here, always wanting to push harder. Additionally, your schedule could conflict with the signs your body is giving off. It's imperative at this time to take a step back and regroup. Do whatever you need to do to become as introspective as possible. The signals your body sends trump any planned schedule.

Listen to Your Body

Listening is a true skill. Sometimes we find it hard to pay attention and listen to a coworker, loved one, or friend. Perhaps we were off daydreaming about something else. Maybe we had a rough day and our mind is spent. It happens; we've all been there. These same challenges exist when you try to listen to yourself, but it can be even trickier because we're not used to doing it. Usually, if we're tired, we go on about our day. If we feel a little sick, we try to go to work anyway. Hopefully, during your TRI training, you can start to catch—and heed—your body's cues and warnings on a more regular basis. It takes some time and focus. Do your best. The added attention to self pays off. Over time, you'll learn when your body is requesting a day off.

Here are some signs that you might need a break in training:

+ Loss of appetite

+ Decrease in performance

+ Abnormal resting heart rate (typically higher than normal)

+ Nagging fatigue

+ Illness

+ Injury

+ Sleep pattern disturbances

+ Lethargy

Heed the Fatigue Warning Signs

It's important to become aware of your body's warning signs and know how they compare with regular fatigue. Then you can apply rest and recovery depending on how efficiently your body processes training loads and external factors.

Some of the categories of fatigue include the following:

◆ Hydration (fatigue from inadequate water replenishment)

◆ Fuel (fatigue from depletion of muscle and liver glycogen)

◆ Lactate production (fatigue from the buildup of lactic acid beyond a certain threshold; primarily associated with pacing at too high of an intensity)

◆ Overtraining (advanced stage of fatigue caused from training beyond your body's ability to cope)

Gains Occur Through Rest

In Chapter 4, we discussed some training principles and introduced the law of overload, which says that beneficial adaptations occur in response to demands placed on the body at levels beyond a certain threshold, but within the limits of tolerance. When we train and place stress on our body, it actually becomes temporarily weakened. Then, during the recovery phase, it rebuilds itself stronger than it was originally. During regeneration, the body overcompensates and you become slightly more fit. The trick becomes stressing your body at loads between your threshold and safe limits.

Coaches' Corner

Steve supplemented his first Ironman training program with yoga. His instructor always talked about pushing your personal limits in class and referred to it as "finding your edge." Each class you could push a position a little farther or hold a position a little longer. The art of TRI training also incorporates this edge. The goal is to exploit the principle of overload until you meet the edge and then back off to allow your body time to absorb the fitness. In other words, quality and consistent training are achieved when you find your edge, learn when to schedule rest, and listen to your body's warning signs.

When your body undergoes training stress, muscles tear, cells break down, and fluid is displaced. A great deal of damage and trauma can take place beneath the surface. If you ever think that recovery isn't that important, think about these physiological effects, and realize that you need to take it seriously.

Overtraining

Overtraining occurs when you pass beyond the edge, to a point where you're not balancing training and recovery. The effects can spread across both physical and psychological domains. We mentioned some of the physical symptoms and warning signs earlier in this chapter. One of the more psychological effects is the inability to concentrate. If you find yourself flirting uncharacteristically with any of these possible effects, take a step back and evaluate yourself and your schedule. Listen to your body. Pay attention to things like your resting heart rate.

If you have a suspicion that you might be overtraining, take a break. We suggest taking 24 to 48 hours of complete rest. Then ease back into an easy workout such as an active recovery session on the bike or a short swim. Keep your heart rate and perceived exertion levels low. If you're still not feeling up to par, repeat the rest period/active recovery workout. It's always better to be safe than sorry when it comes to training. Falling into the abyss of overtraining and trying to rush back to the grind too soon can result in illness, injury, and a great loss in fitness. Remember, consistent training is the key.

Gravel Ahead

Stay away from a whirlpool or hot tub for 24 hours following a difficult workout or race. Heat can be counterproductive when there's swelling (edema) within the body.

Workout Recovery Phases

In addition to straight rest and shortening the duration of your workouts, you can contribute to recovery in other ways. These factors are referred to as workout recovery phases:

- Warm-up
- Fueling during activity
- Cool-down and stretching
- Postactivity fueling
- Sleep

Paying attention to each phase reduces damage while expediting your body's rebuilding process. In other words, when you conduct these phases properly, you recover more quickly.

Warm It Up

A proper warm-up before a workout is like lubing up a dry chain before a bike ride: you become more efficient and decrease your chance of injury. The process gives your body a chance to adapt to an increase in work. Blood moves away from your core and distributes itself appropriately. Heart rate adjusts gradually. Muscles get primed. A good warm-up sets the stage for an efficient recovery process.

Mid-Workout Fueling

During the workout (as discussed in Chapter 9), you should consume calories (fuel). Running your engine on a premium fuel helps your body maximize performance and minimize recovery time. Your performance could drop and the time it took you to feel peppy again might take much longer if you don't fuel during your workout.

Cool It Down

After you finish up a workout, don't forget to cool down. Some newbies want to blow off warm-ups and cool-downs because they want to get right to the meat of the workout. Don't give in to this desire. While a warm-up gets you primed to maximize performance, a cool-down allows your body a chance to redistribute blood, hormones, and other fluids. Give your heart a chance to wind down.

S-T-R-E-T-C-H It Out

Many athletes forget or just leave out stretching because of time. Don't fall into that trap. It's better to cut a workout 5 or 10 minutes short and stretch, than to get the full duration of the activity in and not stretch.

Refuel

After a workout, you need to restore your glycogen stores. Some people choose to kill two birds with one stone by stretching and taking in their postworkout nutrition at the same time. That's fine if you want to combine the two.

Rest Easy

To cap it all off, a good night's sleep after a tough workout helps facilitate a speedy recovery. Growth hormones are released during sleep, which contribute to the fabulous rejuvenation process. Sleep tight, and don't let those bedbugs bite.

Coaches' Corner

Some triathletes augment their recovery using hydrotherapy. You can do this by sitting in cold (or as cool as you can handle) bath water for 5 to 10 minutes. "Cold water?" you say. "How can I relax in that?" The first 30 to 60 seconds are the most difficult but then your body will get used to the temperature and it will actually begin to feel rejuvenating. The science: cold water therapy produces vasoconstriction, which slows circulation, reducing inflammation, muscle spasm, and pain. *Caveat:* hydrotherapy can aggravate some medical conditions, so talk to your doctor before trying this at home.

Rest and recovery are pivotal components to TRI training. That's your time to recharge your batteries. Unfortunately, your body doesn't have an indicator light that turns red when you're running out of juice. You must rely on subtle signals from your mind and body and what you've learned about training and recovery. If you don't make time for recovery, you'll have to make time for illness or injury. We know you'll embrace an R&R plan that works best for you. Stay safe, and train smart.

The Least You Need to Know

- Attitude, motivation, focus, and determination work collaboratively toward setting a solid mind-set.

- Visualizing positive outcomes can help shape your reality.

- Direct your focus to those things you can control.

- Realize that your ego may try to stifle your recovery. Don't let it!

- Build recovery into your schedule, but be ready to work in unplanned recovery when your body sends you signals that it needs it.

- Find your edge, but don't drop over into overtraining.

Part 4

Realizing Your Dream

Triathlon is an exciting and dynamic sport with many variables. Planning is an important factor in the process, as it helps you stay focused. Having a blueprint or road map and applying it to your personal goals is helpful in achieving overall success. Having a goal written down on paper also provides motivation throughout your training.

After training for several weeks or months, your big day will arrive. When you wake up on race day, you will be ready. Do not doubt your ability to train for and complete this triathlon. We give you the tools and help you in every step of the way. Your training teaches you to roll with the punches, so even if something unexpected happens, you won't panic. You'll deal with it and find success—and most likely become addicted to the sport.

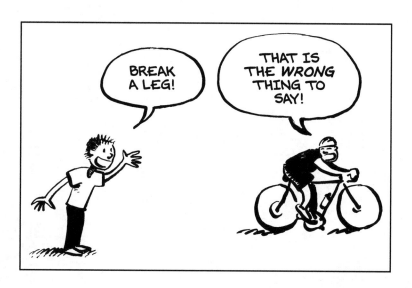

Chapter 12

Scheduling and Tracking Strategies

In This Chapter

◆ What goes into a schedule

◆ How your schedule folds into your life

◆ What to track and how to track it

◆ Understanding TRI programs

We all know time is a precious commodity. The level of commitment necessary to train for a TRI depends on the race distance and your relative fitness level. You need to stay realistic, work with a schedule, and document your progress to help you meet your goals and strike the right balance. Keeping a log of your goals, workouts, races, diet, and rest helps you stay focused and motivated. It also assists in making adjustments to your training regimen and serves as a source of information when you're getting ready for the next TRI.

After you've established a fitness base, using any of the schedules in Chapters 13 and 14 will get you to the finish line of your goal race. You just need to believe in yourself, believe in the program, and put in the time to get the job done. Don't try to fake your way through any of the training plans, especially the ones for longer races. Not only will you miss out on much of the fitness benefits of TRI, but your experience on race day may be less enjoyable, too. Put in the time, and you will find success!

Understanding Workout Schedules

We're going to let you in on a little secret: the most important thing about a training schedule is *not* that it gives you the exact number of minutes or mileage you need to swim, bike, or run on any one day of your training … but simply that it gives you a road map to follow. Many people have many different goals throughout their lives, and unfortunately, many of them never reach their goals. Why? Often the answer is that they don't have a step-by-step process to achieve them. We'll give you that guidance here so you'll never feel lost. Each day, you'll know exactly what to do to train (or rest) your body so you'll be ready to go on race day.

The five training schedules in Chapters 13 and 14 share some like qualities. Each includes swim, bike, and run workouts as well as days to lift weights and stretch. The duration, frequency, and intensity of each vary based on the distance of your goal race, but the overall concepts remain the same.

Another similarity you'll notice is that we schedule the longer bike and run workouts for the weekend, when most people have a little more free time. Feel free to shift the schedule if your free days differ from the standard. Our schedules have a long bike on Saturday and a long run on Sunday, but Steve likes to break up his long bike and run when his schedule permits. He rides long on the weekend and runs long midweek.

> ### Coaches' Corner
>
> It is absolutely okay to tweak your training schedule when necessary. The training plans we give you here are meant to serve as a blueprint. But this isn't an exact science; there's some flexibility.

def•i•ni•tion

> **Periodization** is the blending of workloads, progression, and recovery so optimal fitness gains occur at optimal times. It takes into account all the TRI training principles.

All the programs share a general pattern of building up the minutes you train in each sport from week to week over 3 weeks. Every fourth week is designated a recovery week: the exercise duration of each sport is reduced a bit to allow your body to recover and absorb all the training of the previous weeks. Some find it hard to decrease the amount of training, but gains only occur through rest (remember Chapter 11?). Hopefully you can force yourself to take it down a notch for a week.

The goal of training programs is to apply the concept of *periodization*. One of the objectives of periodization is to build a solid pyramid of fitness using four phases:

- ◆ Preparation
- ◆ Base
- ◆ Build
- ◆ Peak

The other objective is to apply specificity, overload, and reversibility principles in conjunction with frequency, intensity, and duration elements, all while taking into account progression and recovery. Wow, that's a lot of info. Sounds complicated, doesn't it? Don't worry; we guide you through the programs, all of which incorporate these TRI principles. Do your best to follow them, but at the same time, listen to your body and make slight adjustments along the way as necessary.

The Prep Phase

The preparation phase varies based on the distance of your goal race, your aerobic fitness, and your personal abilities. This phase might last for a couple weeks if you've been keeping active before your training program and already have some experience in each of the three disciplines. If you're coming straight from the couch, this phase might take a little longer.

If you feel you're overweight or have any other physical challenges, this is the time to build it up slowly (after getting the okay from a physician, of course). Don't rush through the prep phase just because you're itching to start digging deeper into the training program. Patience is an ally.

If you need some time to work on one (or two or three) of the specific sports, this is the right time to get that done. If the only swimming you know is doggy paddle, work on developing the freestyle (a.k.a., front crawl) during this time.

If your bicycle experience is next to nothing, you might want to get out and ride a couple times a week to get the feel. This is a great idea especially if you'll be using a new type of bike, handlebars, or pedals. If you've added clip or clipless pedals to your arsenal, use this time to become accustomed to generating power in every available direction (not just pushing down on the pedals). If you have a bike trainer available, set up your bike and do some drills (refer to Chapter 6).

The same goes for running. If you haven't run since twelfth-grade PE class, you might want to focus more time on running during the early prep phase. Sometimes it's worth having a specialist take a look at your gait early on. A couple good pointers can save you energy and the risk of injury.

Because of the widely varying backgrounds and needs of different athletes during the prep phase, we don't want to offer a specific program for this. Our advice in this arena is to …

> ### Coaches' Corner
>
> If you're having serious trouble getting the freestyle stroke down, consider taking a private lesson. If you already know the stroke but you feel you aren't improving your speed or efficiency, coached Masters' programs are a good option. Don't be intimidated. You can find a lane that works best for your pace and fitness level.

> ### Training Tips
>
> During your preparation phase, keep FIT (frequency, intensity, time) low. Your heart rate should primarily be in zone 1. This is the time to introduce fitness demands, improve technique, and prepare for the next level—base phase. (See Chapter 4 for more details on F.I.T.)

- Start working out near your current fitness level (i.e., don't try to go out and run 10 miles after not running in years).

- Try to work out three to five times per week, with more workout sessions dedicated to the sport(s) you feel you need the most work in.

- Keep the intensity low, and increase the total minutes per week practiced in each sport by 10 percent.

◆ Progress until you're at the point that you could do the workouts for the first couple weeks of the training program without much difficulty.

Race Options

Remember, you absolutely, positively *do not* have to do a race in your first season, or ever for that matter. Simply training for TRI will bring you most of the fitness and mental benefits. If you do choose to race, you have five major distance options:

◆ Super-sprint   8 week program

◆ Sprint   12 week program

◆ Olympic   16 week program

◆ Half-Ironman   20 week program

◆ Ironman   24 week program

Sprint and Olympic distances are the ones most commonly offered.

Talkin' About TRI

Training for a TRI takes commitment—physical, mental, time, etc. Be sure you work through your goals, time, and expectations with the ones you love. Sit down with your spouse, kids, fiancé, boss, or whomever prior to embarking on the TRI venture. This is a critical element in the overall experience. The more they know and understand up front, the better. You don't want to be halfway through your program and run into conflicts that could have been avoided by talking it through in the beginning.

Your weekly training time can range from 6 to 20 hours a week, depending on what you're training for and where you are in the program. Needless to say, a hefty time and energy commitment is involved. It's important to note that the time commitment is not just the minutes shown on the schedule. For example, a Masters' swim workout might require getting your things together, driving to the pool, changing, the workout, changing back, driving home or to work, etc. A 1-hour swim workout could take 2 hours by the time all's said and done. The same goes for any other session. Keep this in mind as you think through your training capacity.

Gravel Ahead _____

In addition to discussing the time commitment of the sport with friends and family, you should discuss the potential shift in energy. For example, you might be tired after a long bike ride and not feel like getting up early on your day off to get ready for that garage sale. It's important for you to realize your schedule and overall energy level might go through some changes. Discuss these potential issues with those in your life.

Making It All Fit

Time management, creativity, and flexibility—these are the three ingredients that make TRI training efficient. As with anything new, you might have to make a few sacrifices when starting on your TRI training. The level to which these sacrifices occur depends on many variables, such as race distance, career demands, family, current fitness level, etc. You might have to make some trade-offs: a morning run might have to replace reading the morning newspaper with a cup of java; a quick lunch during the work day may be turned into a quick swim at the local pool; happy hour may be postponed by an after-work bike ride.

These little changes can give you a different perspective on life (and some rejuvenating fresh air). Most triathletes welcome the trade-offs that come with the sport.

Time Management

Time management. Important on the job; important in TRI training. You can strategically plan your day to fit in the most stuff in the least amount of time. The end goal is to improve effectiveness and maximize efforts.

How does time management relate to TRI training? We'll show you: your first step on the TRI path is choosing your goal race, using the training programs as a general guideline of how much time you'll need to dedicate to training each week. After you've talked with family and looked at your available capacity, you can set your TRI goal. Then, you can set your sights, get some preparation work out of the way, and use our TRI training schedules to help organize your workouts. You'll be able to see a workout snapshot of the day, week, or month ahead. This serves as the "to-do" list of time management. Keeping your finger on the pulse of the schedule helps you organize each day and stay on track.

Creativity

Unless you're an elite, professional triathlete, you probably have non-TRI things to worry about in your life. Creativity is essential to balance a busy schedule with training. Triathletes must often think outside the box to meet everyday responsibilities while juggling TRI training.

If you find out on Friday afternoon that you have a budget review meeting on Monday and you have a long bike ride scheduled this weekend, you might have to get creative. For example, instead of heading out on the roads for your long bike, you might complete your bike workout indoors on a stationary bike so you can review your budget materials while staying on track with your TRI workout.

Training Tips

It's okay to get creative when approaching your TRI training. In fact, we encourage it. Master this skill, as it helps minimize stress while maximizing performance and overall well-being.

Flexibility

The ability to be flexible with your schedule helps make it all gel. The training plan is a road map, so when life's other commitments conflict with your TRI schedule, you have a couple options. One is to flip-flop days as necessary. If you're traveling on business or pleasure and don't have access to your bike, you can switch your long run day with your long bike workout. If the hotel has a big enough pool, you can hop in and log some minutes in the water.

Another way to work flexibility into your schedule is by reevaluating the hours in your day. Perhaps you were never much of a morning person. Well, that might have to change. Sometimes the only way to meet both TRI and life commitments is by training very early or late, depending on your day.

Training Tips

Getting used to waking up early for training is a good thing, as most races start very early. If a triathlon race has a 7 A.M. start time, you might need to rise as early as 4 A.M., depending on how long it takes to get to the destination and other logistics. Work early morning training into your schedule to help prepare yourself for racing.

Tracking TRI

Logging data from your TRI experience can be a powerful tool. When you track your progress in a diary or other log, you are really able to quantify the progress you make. This data can be used for motivation, guidance, or a benchmark.

When you see the results of your training written down, you really have some motivation in black and white. When you're feeling like you're not progressing, you can look back at your notes for proof. For example, your morning resting heart rate might fall from 70 beats per minute to 55 beats per minute in just a few weeks of training. That knowledge can be a source of energy and drive. Learning to capture and acknowledge these stats can boost your confidence and renew your commitment to training.

Tracking can also provide a sense of guidance. For example, you can look at data to spot trends, such as if working out after 6 P.M. interferes with your sleep. Finding trends or patterns is priceless. You could learn the early signs of burnout, overtraining, or injury and make necessary adjustments before it's too late.

Tracking TRI also serves as a benchmark. It doesn't matter if this is your first race or your fifteenth. You can compare the data you collect with everything you do moving forward. This brings us back to where we started with motivation. A lot of those who get hooked on TRI do it because they want to find their personal best. Tracking your benchmark is just the beginning.

Set Up a Notebook Training Diary

There are no hard-and-fast rules when it comes to developing your training diary method. We outline some options as well as offer some good stats to track. You be the judge on which technique works best for you. You can also mix things up from race to race or year to year until you find the right fit.

Some tracking options you can use include the following:

- The check-off method
- A journal
- A TRI page
- A calendar
- An electronic spreadsheet

> ### Coaches' Corner
>
> We both used a journal to track our TRI progress our first year. Each night, we logged any fitness-related activities we did during the day. Colin also jotted down any nutrition he took in during different workouts, as well as other food he ate throughout the day.

If you think you'll be following one of the training plans in this book to the T, you might choose the check-off method. You can use the training plan as your training journal, dating and checking off each workout as you complete it. You can also make additional notes in the margins to track nutrition or take notes when you deviate slightly from the planned workout.

Using a journal or notebook to keep track of each day is a simple and effective approach to tracking your progress. The journal method is simple to use. All you need is a journal, a pen, and about 10 minutes at the end of each day. One disadvantage: you don't have a quick snapshot of what you've done over more than one day.

Very similar to a journal, you could create a TRI page—a sheet of paper that lists all the statistics you want to keep. Run off multiple copies, bind or staple them, and then fill them out as time goes along. You could type it out and make it fancy or just write it out on a notebook page. You could put only one day on a page or fit in several. This method keeps things organized and consistent (you won't forget which data you're trying to track).

A calendar method entails using a blank calendar page and logging data on each day. Then you can compare what you're doing with the master TRI program. It provides a quick glance of where you are compared with your plan. You do have limited space in each block to outline data, but you can mitigate this by getting an oversized calendar or using a blank page behind each calendar month to catch any information overflow.

> ### Gravel Ahead
>
> If you don't really like the tracking strategy you're using, chances are you *won't* use it. Be sure, when choosing a tracking strategy, to choose one you're comfortable with. If it seems laborious to manage, you're likely to give up. Pick a system you like, and make it part of your daily routine.

For those who have a home computer and a spreadsheet program, you might want to track your progress electronically. This is a great way to document training because there are ways to sort data that would be very difficult to do by hand. Spreadsheet programs can automatically calculate running summaries (total miles), averages (average speed), max and min values (longest distance and fastest pace), etc. If you have a program but aren't sure how to use some of these features, try searching the help feature if you're interested in learning. With a little research and a few minutes to experiment, you could have a spreadsheet to track your progress in no time.

Important Stats

What should you track? Track things like workout modes, intensity, duration, nutrition, and date. Beyond that, several optional choices can only add to your overall TRI learning experience. Some of the stats, like "Average Speed," are shown as a possibility for *bike* data because a bike computer makes the information easy to capture. If you don't have a bike computer, don't go into a lot of trouble to figure out that stat. Remember, the easier and more straight forward your tracking strategy, the more likely you'll be to stick with it.

Here are some suggested stats to log:

- Date*
- Morning heart rate
- Hours slept
- Preworkout fuel
- Workout fuel*
- Postworkout fuel
- Workout(s)*
- Workout time of day
- Conditions: weather/wind

- Heart rate zones
- Duration*
- Location/course*
- Fatigue (scale 1–10) A.M.
- Fatigue (scale 1–10) P.M.
- Workout partner(s)
- Average speed (bike)
- Mileage (bike)/Yardage (swim)
- Comments*

*At a minimum, log this data when you can.

Understanding TRI Programs

Our sprint-distance TRI program (see Chapter 13) is laid out into two main groups: the daily breakdown and the master plan. It begins with the full 12-week plan followed by a step-by-step breakdown of each day. The master plan provides a nice overview of the time you'll spend per day per sport for each phase of training. The daily breakdowns outline clear and concise procedures to follow for each session. In Chapter 14, you'll find master plans, as well as several possible workouts for each race distance.

The programs contain swim, bike, run, weights/stretch, and optional workouts. Swim, bike, and run each have their own category. Some workouts are designated with a T for *Transition* and should be done immediately following the previous sport.

In addition, we have included some *Optional* workouts (O), the majority of which are suggested Saturday swims. These workouts can be done provided you are feeling fresh and up to it.

In Chapter 13, for you more experienced triathletes, we've also worked in degrees of difficulty by tweaking speed, intensity, and recovery. Our daily breakdowns outline ways to make the sessions more challenging. For example, a swim workout may be 60 minutes. However, the distance covered in that fixed time can vary greatly from individual to individual, depending on the pace and rest. TRI Guy Jeff may swim 2,000 yards in a 60-minute period while TRI Gal Missy may swim 3,000 yards in the same period of time because she swims faster and takes less recovery between intervals/sets.

Weights (W) and stretch (S) fall under the *Other* category. We offer little detail in the daily breakdowns for these two aspects, as the regimen won't change much throughout the training program. In Chapter 14, you'll notice that some sets of intervals are designated with a "+" or a "++". That simply means that you should increase your intensity throughout that set. "+" indicates a slight increase; "tt" designates a little bit larger increase.

Keep in mind that the programs are meant to guide you on your TRI journey. You should also leave room for some individual conditions that will influence your schedule.

Coaches' Corner

With weight training, there are a couple schools of thought: some experts and research advocates two or three weight workouts per week during TRI training; others say it's better to focus on TRI-specific training, especially for beginners. We agree that weight training is important for developing power, core strength, and bone density. However, we feel many other variables should be considered: age, current condition, triathlon distance, and time. We covered these factors in greater detail in Chapter 10.

The Least You Need to Know

- TRI programs incorporate periodization—blending training principles to optimize fitness gains.
- Workout schedules provide a road map to help you achieve your TRI goals.
- Receiving support from the important people in your life is an important step in ensuring a smooth TRI experience.
- Learning to incorporate time management skills, creativity, and flexibility helps enhance training.
- Tracking training stats provides a basis for future growth and development.

Chapter 13

TRI a Sprint

In This Chapter

♦ Learning about specific drills in specific sports

♦ Understanding the suggested workouts

♦ A day-by-day sprint training program

Now for the meat and potatoes of this stuff. You've heard the theory. This chapter and the next give you specific workout charts that suggest which sport you should do, for how much time, and on which days. This chapter goes into day by day detail of how to prepare for a sprint-distance TRI.

Because the majority of beginner and intermediate triathletes are training for a sprint triathlon, in this chapter, we give you a day-by-day detailed training schedule for that distance. If you're doing a super-sprint, Olympic, half-Ironman, or Ironman, don't panic! We outline exact workouts, intensities, and suggestions for those programs in the next chapter.

Z1? 4×50? What's This All Mean?

The daily schedule is pretty straightforward, but we want to be sure you understand what you're reading. At the most basic level, we use numbers to show how many sets and repetitions (reps) of different exercises are suggested. For instance:

8×2-minute intervals at Z3 (1 minute recovery)

This means to do a 2-minute interval, during which you should be working hard enough so your heart rate is in zone 3 (Z3; measured either with a heart rate monitor or by perceived exertion). At the end of the 2-minute interval, you back off the pace and recover for 1 minute. You then repeat the entire process 7 more times for a total of 8. Make sense?

Below certain workouts, we've added an asterisk (*) and suggestions for how a more advanced triathlete could increase the volume or intensity of a designated workout. Even if you consider yourself a more advanced triathlete, don't feel like you have to adjust your workout with these suggestions. Always, always, always do what is right for you.

Swim Notes

Swim workouts are described in minutes as well as in distance. The duration is an estimate because different swimmers complete the workout in different amounts of time. If you reach the designated time before you complete the workout, you can cut yourself off at that point after you do a cool-down. If you go over the designated time to complete the workout, it won't negatively impact your training.

Additionally, we didn't put a unit of measure on the distances, as some pools are measured in meters and some in yards. These two distances are similar, so you can just use the numbers in the workout descriptions and assume we meant the unit by which your pool is measured. The final number shown marked as "Total" combines all the distances that make up the warm-up, workout, and cool-down … again, in the unit of measure of your pool.

> ### Coaches' Corner
>
> At most pools, the length of a lap lane is 25 meters or 25 yards. If the distance across your pool is different, don't panic! The most important aspect of the workout is the amount of time you spend swimming. Adjust the workouts as necessary to fit your pool's length. If possible, try to find a pool that is at least 20 meters or 20 yards long so you have enough room to stretch out your form.

Bike Notes

Some bike workouts are described for athletes using an indoor trainer. You can try to do some of the suggested workouts on the road, but if you do, be sure you do it in an area with very little to no traffic. Do not attempt the single leg drills (SLD) out on the road, as it could cause you to lose balance. If you don't have a trainer, we generally suggest skipping the big gear drills (BGD)/small gear drills (SGD)/SLD workouts and completing hill intervals on that day.

Also, unless otherwise noted, your cadence on the bike should be somewhere between 80 and 100 RPMs. We let you know when to adjust it.

Weight Lifting and Stretching Notes

We've put two suggested sessions of weight lifting and one suggested session of stretching in most weeks of each training plan. As discussed in Chapter 12, adjust the placement of these sessions as necessary. There are many schools of thought on weight lifting and stretching as related to TRI. Follow your common sense or your doctor's orders, or get some personal advice from a mentor. We won't discuss either in the day-to-day descriptions; however, refer to Chapter 10 for further details on weight training and flexibility.

Zone Notes

Whether you're wearing a heart rate monitor or using your rate of perceived exertion, we designate the level at which you should be pushing yourself in the daily descriptions and in the workout chart at the end of the chapter. But instead of writing out "… in Zone 1" or "… at 60 percent of your max heart rate" or "… in an active recovery zone," we use abbreviations.

Levels of Exertion

Description	Zone	Percent of Max Heart Rate	RPE	Abbreviation
Active recovery	1	55 to 65	12 to 13	Z1
Endurance	2	65 to 75	13 to 15	Z2
Resistance	3	75 to 85	15 to 16	Z3
Threshold	4	85 to 90	16 to 18	Z4

One Last Thing

We list the days as Day 1, Day 2, Day 3, … Day 7 for every week. The eventual race will land on Day 7, so we consider Day 6 and Day 7 the weekend (most races occur on Sundays). As mentioned earlier, you should feel free to move around any of the workouts. Want to shift the entire program over on the calendar so that, for instance, Day 1 is a Wednesday and Day 7 is a Tuesday? Do it. Make the program work for you.

Sprint!

This program is 12 weeks long and is a great place to enter the world of TRI because most local events include a race of this distance. In your preparation phase, you should have built up to the following durations:

◆ Swim: 20 to 25 minutes

◆ Bike: 40 to 45 minutes

◆ Run: 30 to 35 minutes

With the biking, you should try to get to the point where you can ride for 40 minutes without stopping. With the swimming and running, nonstop activity would be good if possible, but don't worry if you need to rest on the wall during a swim session or walk during a run workout. Almost every one of our swim sessions has rest time built in anyway!

Coaches' Corner

Remember, there is no exact science to a training program. What might work perfectly for your friend might not work at all for you. The programs in this book are meant to be guidelines, not the end-all, be-all, for your training. Allow yourself flexibility if your life's schedule gets too hectic. More importantly, listen to your body and adjust your program based on how you feel. Use common sense at all times, and you'll be fine.

Week 1

Date: _____

Day 1   As this is your first official day of training, start off easy with a 20-minute swim. Don't stress yourself out if you don't finish the full distance. Do your best, and just be sure you get a cool-down in at the end.

Swim:

Warm-up	4×50 nice and easy (15 seconds rest)
Workout	6×75 at Z2 (15 seconds rest)
Cool-down	6×25 nice and easy (10 seconds rest)
TOTAL	800

* Increase each workout rep length by 25: workout = 6×100 at Z2 (TOTAL: 950).

Day 2   Hopefully you prepared well enough that your shoulders aren't sore from yesterday's swim. Today you'll just do a simple run of 30 minutes. Nothing fancy, just go out and keep it steady in Z1 or Z2.

Day 3   Take an easy spin of 45 minutes out on the road (or on the indoor trainer if the weather isn't conducive).

Day 4   Get back in the pool again. This time we'll add a little time/distance (25 minutes total).

Swim:

Warm-up	5×50 nice and easy (15 seconds rest)
Workout	6×100 at Z2 (15 seconds rest)
Cool-down	6×25 nice and easy (10 seconds rest), as alternating swim/drill (i.e., your first 25 is done as swimming freestyle, the next 25 is done as a drill of your choice, then 25 freestyle, and so on)
TOTAL	1,000

* Increase warm-up by 1 rep, increase workout rep length by 2 reps, and decrease rest times by 5 seconds (TOTAL: 1,250).

Day 5   Take a break! Don't do anything physical today. You've just completed 4 days in a row of this TRI training program, and your body needs a short break. Because this is only the first week of training, you probably won't feel like you *need* the rest … but resist the urge to go work out.

Day 6   You have your first transition workout today, and if you've never done one before, it'll probably feel a little strange. That's normal, and that's also why we're doing it today (and during many training sessions): so it won't feel strange during your race. Set up all the gear you need for your run and then head out on your bike.

Bike: 45-minute bike, nice and easy (Z1 or Z2). Try to do it at a time when there isn't too much traffic on the road. On the weekends, earlier is generally better.

Run: T-run! Do this 10-minute run right after you finish your bike ride (Z1). It's perfectly fine to grab an energy bar or drink, but don't dawdle too long. Try to get out the door in a few minutes (ideally within 5 to 10). You might find that it's difficult to keep your heart rate or breathing under control when you start the run. Slow down, and take it easy. Just try to get the feel of running off the bike.

Swim (optional): After you finish your bike/run workout and get an opportunity to stretch and refuel, take a break. Later, if you have some energy in reserve, hop in the pool and go for a very short swim (no more than 15 minutes). Take it easier than easy. You shouldn't be breathing hard at any point during this workout. You can swim laps, practice your drills, or see how far you can swim underwater. Have fun and keep it loose.

Day 7   Traditionally, this will be our long run day. In this first week, the run is only 7 minutes longer than our Day 2 run, but that gap will widen as time goes on. Keep it nice and easy as you head out today for a 37-minute run.

Week 2

Date: _____

Day 1   We keep the duration the same as last week's Day 4 swim (25 minutes). Again, don't worry about it if the time it takes you to complete the workout doesn't exactly match what's here. It's more important right now to focus on the total time. Make slight adjustments to get it in—including the cool-down.

Swim:

Warm-up	4×50 nice and easy (15 seconds rest)
Workout	10×50 at Z2 (15 seconds rest); 10×25 at Z2 high (10 seconds rest)
Cool-down	2×100 nice and easy (10 seconds rest)
TOTAL	1,000

* *Do 16×50 as main set (no 25s) (TOTAL: 1,200).*

Day 2   Head out for a steady 35-minute run. If this is only your second week of running, keep it nice and easy.

If you've got a strong background in running or if you have built a solid base in the past several weeks and feel very comfortable with running, you might want to introduce a little speed work. Only consider this if you've already been running for several weeks and last week's run workouts were no problem.

Run:

Warm-up	15 minutes nice and easy
Workout	10 minutes of pick-ups, alternating 1 minute faster, 1 minute recovery (faster minutes should be at Z2 high/Z3); the fast minutes are not all-out sprints, just an increase in speed
Cool-down	5 to 10 minutes easy

Day 3   Just like last week, put in 45 minutes on your metal steed.

Day 4   We don't increase the workout very much today, so it should end up similar to the past two in duration (25 minutes).

Swim:

Warm-up	6×50 nice and easy (15 seconds rest)
Workout	2×150 at Z2 (15 seconds rest); 3×100 at Z2 (10 seconds rest)
Cool-down	4×50 nice and easy (10 seconds rest)
TOTAL	1,100

* For workout, do 6×150 (no 100s) and decrease rest times by 5 seconds (TOTAL: 1,250).

Day 5   Take a break, triathlete!

Day 6   After your long bike today, do another T-run. Hopefully, it feels more natural this week. Remember to set up all the gear you need for your run before you head out on your bike.

Bike: 55-minute bike, nice and easy (Z1 or Z2). Set the alarm early to avoid traffic.

Run: T-run! Do this 10-minute run right after you finish your bike ride (Z1). Like last week, try to get out the door in a few minutes, but don't rush too much. Keep your heart rate and breathing under control by keeping the pace easy.

Swim (optional): If you have the energy, you can practice your drills or do a few laps for about 15 minutes. If you get to the pool and feel like just laying in the sun or poolside, that's fine, too.

Day 7   Your long run increases by 3 minutes (40 minutes) from last week. Keep the pace relaxed, and utilize the "talk test" to be sure you're not pushing too hard.

Week 3

Date: _____

Day 1 25 minutes should be old hat by this point …

Swim:

Warm-up	2×100 nice and easy (15 seconds rest) as 100 swim, 100 drill
Workout	7×100 at Z2 (20 seconds rest)
Cool-down	4×50 nice and easy (10 seconds rest)
TOTAL	1,100

* Increase workout set to 9 reps and decrease rest by 5 seconds (TOTAL: 1,300).

Day 2 If running is very new to you, just go out and keep it steady in Z1 or Z2 for 35 minutes. Don't start speed work until Week 5.

If you're comfortable with the speed work, then keep it up … and today, add some accelerations and drills. We suggest doing the accelerations between your warm-up and your workout. At that point your legs are ready for action, and the accelerations (which are relatively short) prepare them for the upcoming speed training.

Run:

Warm-up	10 minutes nice and easy; 4 accelerations
Workout	15 minutes of intervals as 3×2 minute intervals, with 3 minutes recovery between (faster minutes should be at Z2 high/Z3 low)
Drills	1×25 per leg of each drill
Cool-down	10 minutes easy

Day 3 If you're still getting used to your bike, just go out for a nice 45-minute ride. If you're feeling really comfortable in the saddle, do your first speed workout on the bike today. Do some intervals to see how you feel with bike speed.

Bike:

Warm-up	15 minutes nice and easy
Workout	20 minutes of intervals as 4×3 minute intervals, with 2 minutes recovery between (faster minutes should be at Z2 high/Z3 low. If you don't feel like you have enough recovery time between intervals, you're probably pushing too hard during the interval; crank it down a notch.)
Cool-down	10 minutes easy

Day 4 Up your time in the pool by about 5 minutes to 30 minutes today.

Swim:

Warm-up	3×100 nice and easy (15 seconds rest)
Workout	8×50 at Z2 (10 seconds rest); 4×100 at Z2 (15 seconds rest)
Cool-down	4×50 nice and easy (10 seconds rest)
TOTAL	1,300

* For workout, do 8×100 and 4×50 (TOTAL: 1,500).

Day 5 Kick back and relax.

Day 6 You know the Day 6 drill: long bike/T-run/optional swim. Try to learn from each T-run and improve your transition setup and pace each week.

Bike: 65-minute bike, nice and easy (Z1 or Z2). Now that you're breaking the 1-hour mark, be sure to bring along some sort of hydration and possibly some food (better to have too much than too little).

Run: T-run! Is this 10-minute run (Z1) starting to feel natural?

Swim (optional): Drills? Laps? Diving for pennies?

Day 7 Your relaxed, long run increases by 5 minutes from last week to 45 minutes. Remember, it's okay to take a break and walk if necessary.

Week 4

Date: _____

You'll notice that the durations of most of the workouts go down during this recovery week. Give your body time to rebuild. Less is more.

Day 1 Get wet and take it easy. The distance and time decrease a bit this week (20 minutes).

Swim:

Warm-up	4×50 nice and easy (15 seconds rest)
Workout	6×75 at Z2 (15 seconds rest)
Cool-down	6×25 nice and easy (10 seconds rest)
TOTAL	800

* Increase each workout rep length by 25 (TOTAL: 950).

Day 2 Running is relatively new to you? Do an easy 30-minute run.

You were born to run? Do a fartlek, and only push yourself when you feel like it. Try to stay anywhere below Z4 when you're picking up the pace.

Run:

Warm-up	10 minutes nice and easy; 4 accelerations
Workout	15 minutes of fartlek (pick up and back off the pace whenever you feel like it)
Drills	1×25 per leg of each drill
Cool-down	10 minutes easy

Day 3 If you skipped the intervals last week, don't start them until next week; do a 35-minute ride. If you did the speed work in week 3, get back on that horse and do some intervals.

Bike:

Warm-up	10 minutes nice and easy
Workout	15 minutes of intervals as 3×3 minute intervals, with 2 minutes recovery between (faster minutes should be at Z2 mid to high)
Cool-down	10 minutes easy

Day 4 Like Day 1 of this week, back off the time and distance a bit (25 minutes).

Swim:

Warm-up	6×50 nice and easy (15 seconds rest)
Workout	5×50 at Z2 high (15 seconds rest); 10×25 at Z3 (10 seconds rest)
Cool-down	2×100 nice and easy (15 seconds rest)
TOTAL	1,000

* Do 20×50 as main set (no 25s) (TOTAL: 1,250).

Day 5 Watch a movie, read a book, or surf the web … just don't exercise today.

Day 6 The long bike isn't as long today, and no swim is on the calendar. After your T-run, take the afternoon off.

Bike: 50-minute bike, nice and easy (Z1 or Z2).

Run: T-run! 10 minutes; your legs should be used to it by now.

Day 7 Reel back the long run by 10 minutes this week, in honor of the recovery gods; 35 minutes on the trails, road, or treadmill.

Week 5

Date: _____

Day 1   Do you know why you should be excited? Today is your first transition-bike workout! After your 30-minute swim, hop on your bike and ride around for about 10 minutes to get the feel for that transition.

Swim:

Warm-up	5×50 nice and easy (15 seconds rest) as drill/pull/drill/kick/drill
Workout	3×100 at Z2 (15 seconds rest), 3×200 at Z2 (25 seconds rest)
Cool-down	2×100 nice and easy (10 seconds rest)
TOTAL	1,350

* Increase 200s and decrease 100s, 1 for 1 (e.g., 2×100, 4×200) up to 7×200 (TOTAL potential: 1,650).

Bike: Your first T-bike! Ride nice and easy for 10 minutes to get comfortale pedaling fresh out the water.

Day 2   Everyone should be on the speedwork bandwagon after today! Be confident in your ability, and get it done. The workout should take about 35 minutes.

Run:

Warm-up	15 minutes nice and easy; 6 accelerations
Workout	10-minute tempo run (Your pace should be a bit challenging, but not quite as fast as interval speed; try to keep it in Z2 high/Z3 low.)
Drills	1×25 per leg of each drill
Cool-down	10 minutes easy

Day 3   If you have an indoor trainer, set up your bike and get ready for a 40-minute drill workout.

Bike:

Warm-up	15 minutes nice and easy
Workout	4×30 seconds SLD (see Chapter 6 for info on drills) trying to focus on the full rotation of the pedal (i.e., your power should *not* just be coming from the downstroke); 2 minutes easy in normal cadence; 5×2 minutes of LGD with 1 minute recovery between (LGD should be at a cadence at least 20 RMPs slower than your normal, in a very hard gear)
Cool-down	10 minutes easy

If you don't have an indoor trainer, try to find a pretty steep hill to ride up. Do 4 minutes uphill (hard), 2 minutes downhill, and repeat 3 times. When going uphill, your heart rate will spike. Pace yourself and try not to let your heart rate get too high.

Day 4   Up your time in the pool by about 5 minutes to 35 minutes today.

Swim:

Warm-up	3×100 nice and easy (15 seconds rest)
Workout	10×50 at Z3 (10 seconds rest); 5×100 at Z3 (15 seconds rest) (It will be hard to catch your breath during this workout if you're really in Z3, but push through it. Even as you get fatigued, try to focus on keeping good form.)
Cool-down	4×50 nice and easy (10 seconds rest)
TOTAL	1,500 yards

* For workout, add 5 more 50s to the set (total of 15), and decrease the rest for the 100s to 10 seconds (TOTAL: 1,750).

Day 5   Ahhh … day 5 decompression.

Day 6   Try to bike somewhere new during your 70-minute ride today. If you decide to drive yourself to a new location, be sure to bring gear for your T-run. *Bike:* 70-minute bike, in Z1 or Z2. Adjust your hydration/nutrition plan based on what you've learned in the past month.

Run: T-run! A little longer this week (15 minutes), but it shouldn't cause you any problems. Take it nice and slow, (Z1).

Swim (optional): Short and easy!

Day 7   Your relaxed, long run is the same duration as Week 3 (45 minutes). Employ the talk test to be sure you're keeping it aerobic. Oxygen is good.

Week 6

Date: _____

Sometime this week, try to work in an open-water swim if possible. Go to your local beach with a buddy, and see what it's like when you're swimming with waves and current, without walls or crystal clear water. When you're out there, just swim for time and don't worry about the distance. We put the suggestion in there a few times this week; pick the one that works with your schedule.

Day 1   35 minutes of swimming, same duration as last week's Day 4.

Warm-up	6×50 nice and easy (15 seconds rest)
Workout	6×100 at Z2 (15 seconds rest); 2×200 at Z2 (20 seconds rest)
Cool-down	5×50 nice and easy (15 seconds rest)
TOTAL	1,550

* For workout, add a 200 and decrease the rest for the 100s to 10 seconds (TOTAL: 1,750).

Day 2   Run 35 minutes. We feel the need for speed! Enjoy the intervals. Before or after your run workout, you might want to fit in an open-water swim.

Run:

Warm-up	10 minutes nice and easy, 6 accelerations
Workout	15-minute set of intervals; 2 minutes pickup, 1 minute easy (pickups in Z2 high/Z3 low)
Drills	1×25 per leg of each drill (increase to 2×20 if you feel like it)
Cool-down	10 minutes easy

Swim (optional): 12 to 20 minutes of open-water swimming with a partner. Be safe!

Day 3   Bike 50 minutes. If you have an indoor trainer, find something fun on TV and hit these drills. We have an optional T-run on the schedule that can be done after your bike workout if you're feeling up to it. Before or after your bike workout, you might want to fit in an open-water swim.

Bike:

Warm-up	15 minutes nice and easy
Workout	6×30 seconds SLD trying to focus on the full rotation of the pedal; 2 minutes easy in normal cadence; 5×2 minutes of LGD with 1 minute recovery between (Large Gear interval should be at a cadence at least 20 RMPs slower than your normal, in a very hard gear.)
Cool-down	10 minutes easy

If you don't have an indoor trainer, hit the hills. Do 4 minutes uphill (hard), 2 minutes downhill, and repeat 4 times. Watch that heart rate!

Run (optional): 10-minute T-run after this bike workout. If you're up to it, include short T-runs after all your Day 3 bike workouts from here on out.

Swim (optional): 12 to 20 minutes of open-water swimming with a partner. Be safe! Better to err on the side of caution with regards to time, as there isn't a wall to hang onto in the open water.

Day 4   40 minutes in the water today. The swim portion of your triathlon won't take nearly this long, but these workouts will prepare you for the big day.

Swim:

Warm-up	3×100 nice and easy (15 seconds rest)
Workout	8×50 at Z3 (10 seconds rest); 5×100 descending pace (faster with each consecutive 100) with 15 seconds rest; 2×200 at Z2 with 20 seconds rest

Cool-down	2×100 nice and easy (10 seconds rest)
TOTAL	1,800 yards

* For workout, add an extra 100 and an extra 200 (TOTAL: 2,100).

Day 5 Rest up.

Day 6 Long bike and T-run and possibly an open-water swim …

Bike: 82-minute bike, in Z1 or Z2. Don't forget your fluids and energy.

Run: T-run! Do this 15-minute run right after you finish your bike ride (Z1).

Swim (optional): Short and easy; practice your drills or do a few laps. Or work in 12 to 20 minutes of open-water swimming with a partner. Be safe!

Day 7 50 minutes on the road. Stay comfortable; breathe easy.

Week 7

Date: _____

Day 1 40 minutes of swimming, same duration as last week's Day 4.

Warm-up	3×100 nice and easy (20 seconds rest)
Workout	6×200 at Z2 (25 seconds rest)
Cool-down	6×50 nice and easy (10 seconds rest)
TOTAL	1,800 yards

* For workout, add a 200 and decrease the rest by 5 seconds (TOTAL: 2,000).

Day 2 Feel the need, the need for speed! Longer intervals today, but the ratio of recovery/interval has gone up, too (35 minutes).

Run:

Warm-up	10 minutes nice and easy; 4 accelerations (longer than normal)
Workout	15-minute set of intervals; 3×3 minutes pickup, 2 minutes easy between (pickups in Z2 high/Z3 low)
Drills	2×20 per leg of each drill
Cool-down	10 minutes easy

Day 3 Bike 55 minutes. Set up the indoor trainer if you've got one.

Bike:

Warm-up	15 minutes nice and easy
Workout	4×1 minutes SGD fast spinning (don't bounce in your seat!); start the first 1 minute rep at 5 RPM faster than your normal cadence;

increase the cadence with each successive minute; 1-minute recovery between; 5×2 minutes of LGD with 1-minute recovery between (Large Gear interval should be at a cadence at least 20 RPMs slower than your normal, in a very hard gear); 4×1 minutes SGD fast spinning

Cool-down	10 minutes easy

If you don't have an indoor trainer, try to find 5×4 minute hill repeats.

Run: Although it's not on the schedule, you can do an optional 10-minute T-run after this bike workout (and after every bike workout).

Day 4 Jump in and swim for 40 minutes.

Swim:

Warm-up	3×100 nice and easy (15 seconds rest)
Workout	8×50 at Z3 (10 seconds rest); 5×100 descending pace (faster with each consecutive 100) with 15 seconds rest; 3×200 at Z2 with 20 seconds rest
Cool-down	2×100 nice and easy (10 seconds rest)
TOTAL	1,800

* For workout, add an extra 100 and an extra 200 (TOTAL: 2,100).

Day 5 Take a break before your longest bike ride of the program.

Day 6 Longest bike ride of the program! Followed by … you guessed it … a T-run.

Bike: 90-minute bike, in Z1 or Z2. Don't forget your fluids and energy.

Run: T-run! Do this 15-minute run right after you finish your bike ride (Z1).

Swim (optional): Short and easy; practice your drills or do a few laps. The schedule says 15 minutes, but feel free to stay in the pool a while longer if you're feeling up to it.

Day 7 We hope it is a beautiful day for a 55-minute run.

Week 8

Date: _____

Your goal this week is to let your body recover. Put in your time, but don't try to be a hero!

Day 1 Rein it in a bit: we'll only be in the pool for 30 minutes today.

Swim:

Warm-up	6×50 nice and easy (15 seconds rest) as swim/pull/drill/swim/pull/drill

Workout	4×100 at Z2 (15 seconds rest), 3×200 at Z2 (25 seconds rest)
Cool-down	4×50 nice and easy (10 seconds rest)
TOTAL	1,500

* Increase 200s and decrease 100s, 1 for 1 (e.g., 3×100, 4×200) up to 7×200 (TOTAL potential: 1,900).

Day 2   Today's tempo run should be just that: a good tempo; a nice pace. Don't go out there and sprint. Keep it steady throughout. You'll run for 30 minutes, but the drills will add a little extra time.

Run:

Warm-up	10 minutes nice and easy, 6 accelerations
Workout	10-minute tempo run in Z2 high/Z3 low
Drills	2×25 per leg of each drill
Cool-down	10 minutes easy

Day 3   Today: a 50-minute bike workout on the streets. Although we don't have it on the schedule, feel free to do a 10-minute T-run after the bike.

Bike:

Warm-up	15 minutes nice and easy
Workout	5 intervals of 3 minutes at Z3; 2 minutes easy in between
Cool-down	10 minutes easy

* Increase interval length to 4 minutes and reduce recovery to 1 minute.

Day 4   Splish, splash you were taking a swim! 30 minutes in the wet.

Warm-up	2×100 nice and easy (15 seconds rest) as swim/pull/drill
Workout	10×100 at Z2 (15 seconds rest)
Cool-down	4×50 nice and easy (10 seconds rest)
TOTAL	1,400

* Do 7×200 instead of 10×100; keep rest at 15 seconds (TOTAL: 1,800).

Day 5   Rest day in a recovery week. What could be more relaxing?

Day 6   Really scale back the long bike this week, and cut the T-run a bit.

Bike: 60-minute bike, in Z1 or Z2.

Run: T-run! Have you had your "transition area" setup just right in previous weeks? Constantly tweak it until you've got it exactly as you want it. Do 10 minutes in Z1 after the bike.

Swim (optional): Short and easy; practice your drills or do a few laps. The schedule says 15 minutes, but feel free to stay in the pool a while longer if you're feeling up to it.

Day 7 40 minutes on the road should seem relatively short today. Don't go all out just because the run is a little shorter.

Week 9

T minus 4 weeks until race day. Start to get focused on that end goal!

Date: _____

Day 1 40 *minutos en el agua.*

Swim:

Warm-up	3×100 nice and easy (15 seconds rest) as drill/pull
Workout	4×300 at Z2 (30 seconds rest)
Cool-down	6×50 nice and easy (10 seconds rest)
TOTAL	1,800 yards

> ** For workout, add a 300 and decrease the rest by 5 seconds (TOTAL: 2,100).*

Day 2 Intervals are integral! It should take you about 35 minutes today (not including the drill time).

Run:

Warm-up	10 minutes nice and easy, 6 accelerations
Workout	15-minutes of intervals as 6×2 with 30 seconds recovery; you will be out of breath, but keep your pickups below Z4
Drills	2×30 per leg of each drill
Cool-down	10 minutes easy

> ** Increase pickups to 3 minutes, and give yourself 45 seconds to recover.*

Day 3 Set up the indoor trainer and start spinning. It should take you about 50 minutes.

Bike:

Warm-up	15 minutes nice and easy
Workout	5×1 minute SGD fast spinning (don't bounce in your seat!); start the first 1 minute rep at 5 RPM faster than your normal cadence; increase the cadence with each successive minute; 1 minute recovery between; 2×2 minutes of LGD with 1 minute recovery between (BGD interval should be at a cadence at least 20 RPMs

slower than your normal, in a very hard gear); 5×1 minute SGD fast spinning; try to keep in Z3 mid to Z4 low for all intervals

| Cool-down | 10 minutes easy |

If you don't have an indoor trainer, try to do two long intervals on the road. After the warm-up, do a 10-minute interval in Z3 mid to Z4 low, recover for 5 minutes, and do another 10-minute interval at Z3 mid/Z4 low.

Run: 10-minute T-run if you want.

Day 4 Lucky 7s! It should take you about 40 minutes.

Swim:

Warm-up	3×100 nice and easy (15 seconds rest)
Workout	7×100 at Z3 low (15 seconds rest); easy 100; 7×50 at Z3 mid/high (10 seconds rest); easy 100; 7×25 descending pace at Z4 (5 seconds rest) (You'll be winded, but concentrate on keeping good form.)
Cool-down	300 nice and easy; take a break if you need to
TOTAL	2,025 yards

*For workout, make it Lucky 9s and try to make each consecutive rep within a given set faster (TOTAL: 2,375).

Day 5 Hopefully you'll feel like you really need that break after yesterday's hard swim.

Day 6 Long bike/T-run.

Bike: 75-minute bike, in Z1 or Z2. Don't forget your fluids and energy.

Run: T-run! Do this 10-minute (minimum) run right after you finish your bike ride (Z1).

Swim (optional): Short and easy; practice your drills or do a few laps. The schedule says 15 minutes, but feel free to stay in the pool a while longer if you're feeling up to it.

Day 7 Your longest run of the program: 60 minutes. Stay aerobic.

Week 10

Date: _____

You'll notice that some of the workouts are getting shorter at this point, but the intensity is still way up there on the days when you're doing speed work.

Day 1 40 minutes of pool time. Today's workout includes some really long intervals. Keep them aerobic. Use the time to monitor your form and make adjustments as necessary. If the race you're training for has a 750 meter swim, you might want to do 350-800-350 instead of 3×500.

Swim:

Warm-up	8×25 nice and easy (5 seconds rest) (Try to decrease the number of strokes it takes you to cross the pool with each consecutive length.)
Workout	3×500 at Z2 (60 seconds rest)
Cool-down	6×50 nice and easy (10 seconds rest)
TOTAL	2,000

For workout, add a fast 50 (Z3) between the 500s (500-50-500-50-500) and decrease the rest by 20 seconds (TOTAL: 2,100).

Run: T-run 10 minutes in Z1.

Day 2   Feel like a fartlek? Go do it for 35 minutes.

Run:

Warm-up	10 minutes nice and easy, 8 accelerations
Workout	15-minute fartlek, trying to keep the pickups in Z3/4 low
Drills	2×30 per leg of each drill
Cool-down	10 minutes easy

Day 3   Indoor trainer? Clipless pedals? Set up your bike and get ready for some drills for 45 minutes. Again, no T-run on the schedule, but you can decide to go the extra mile … literally.

Bike:

Warm-up	15 minutes nice and easy
Workout	5×4 minutes, with the 4 minutes consisting of 1 minute LGD, 1 minute SGD fast spinning, 1 minute of SLD (30 seconds each leg), 1 minute recovery; focus on your form; use the full pedal rotation to apply force in every direction; Z3/4
Cool-down	10 minutes easy

For those without the indoor trainer, hit the hills.

Day 4   Swim 40 minutes. Speed and some distance in the water today.

Swim:

Warm-up	3×100 nice and easy (15 seconds rest)
Workout	Repeat this 3 times: 3×75 at Z3 high/Z4 with 1×250 at Z2 mid/Z3 low to cap it off (15 seconds rest)

Cool-down	300 nice and easy; take a break if you need to
TOTAL	2,025 yards

For workout, add an extra set of 75s at the end (TOTAL: 2,250).

Day 5 Spend some time with your loved ones … unless they're out training for their own race ….

Day 6 Long bike/T-run.

Bike: 65-minute bike, in Z1 or Z2. Don't forget your fluids and energy.

Run: T-run 10 minutes in Z1. Increase the duration if you feel like it.

Swim (optional): Short and easy; drills or laps, or just lay on a raft in the pool.

Day 7 50 minutes in the running shoes. As always: aerobic.

Week 11

Date: _____

Begin the taper this week. Although we haven't been specifically mentioning weight lifting, if you've been doing it, now is the time to stop. You can start up again after your race.

Day 1 Only 35 minutes in the water today.

Swim:

Warm-up	2×100 nice and easy (15 seconds rest)
Workout	6×100 at Z3 mid (15 seconds rest); 3×200 at Z2 (25 seconds rest)
Cool-down	4×50 nice and easy (15 seconds rest)
TOTAL	1,600 yards

For workout, add a 200 and decrease the rest for the 100s to 10 seconds (TOTAL: 1,800).

Day 2 When you run, does the beat of your feet give you a good rhythm? What song runs through your head? Hopefully it has a good *tempo* and you can repeat it for 30 minutes.

Run:

Warm-up	10 minutes nice and easy, 5 accelerations
Workout	10-minute tempo run; try to go for the 10 minutes at race pace (if you're not sure, make your best guess); keep your heart rate out of Z4
Drills	2×15 per leg of each drill
Cool-down	10 minutes easy

Day 3 Skip the indoor trainer. Head outdoors for this week's bike workout of 45 minutes. Go for a T-run after the bike if you feel like it.

Bike:

Warm-up	15 minutes nice and easy
Workout	Intervals of 4×3 minutes hard/2 minutes recovery; intervals should be in Z3/4 (As you probably know by now, going up a hill during the interval helps get your heart rate up quickly.)
Cool-down	10 minutes easy

Day 4 30 minutes of swimming. Speed and some distance in the water today.

Swim:

Warm-up	4×100 nice and easy (15 seconds rest) as kick/pull/drill/swim
Workout	16×50 descending speed, starting at Z2 low and ending at Z4 (10 seconds rest)
Cool-down	6×50 nice and easy (10 seconds rest)
TOTAL	1,500 yards

*Add 4 50s to the workout (TOTAL: 1,700).

Day 5 Rest up! That's an order.

Day 6 Long bike/T-run.

Bike: 55-minute bike, in Z1 or Z2. Don't forget your fluids and energy.

Run: T-run in Z1. 10 minutes.

Swim (optional): Short and easy; drills or laps.

Day 7 Only 40 minutes this week.

Week 12

Date: _____

Race week is finally here! Now you *really* decrease the durations.

Day 1 Only 30 minutes at the pool today.

Swim:

Warm-up	2×100 nice and easy (15 seconds rest)
Workout	3×100 at Z3 mid (20 seconds rest); 4×200 at Z2 (25 seconds rest)

Cool-down	4×50 nice and easy (10 seconds rest)
TOTAL	1,500

For workout, add a 200 and decrease the rest for the 100s to 15 seconds (TOTAL: 1,700).

Day 2 With the duration coming down to only 25 minutes, there isn't much time for the speedwork … but you can get it in there.

Run:

Warm-up	10 minutes nice and easy, 4 accelerations
Workout	5×30 seconds fast (Z3 mid to Z4 low), 1 minute easy between
Drills	1×20 per leg of each drill
Cool-down	7.5 minutes easy

Day 3 Skip the trainer again, and get outside for some quick intervals during this 45-minute bike workout.

Bike:

Warm-up	15 minutes nice and easy
Workout	Intervals of 4×2 minutes as hard/fast spin/hard/fast spin, all with 3 minutes recovery between; intervals should be in Z3/4.
Cool-down	10 minutes easy

Run: 10-minute T-run if you want.

Day 4 Around 30 minutes today, but feel free to cut out a couple of reps here or there if you want to get a little more rest.

Swim:

Warm-up	2×100 nice and easy (15 seconds rest) as swim/choice/swim
Workout	1×200 Z2, 2×100 Z2 high, 3×75 Z3 low, 4×50 Z3 high, 5×25 Z4 high (15 seconds rest)
Cool-down	5×50 nice and easy (10 seconds rest)
TOTAL	1,500 yards

Day 5 Rest up. That's an order.

Day 6 Short workouts of everything today to get your muscles loose after your rest day. If possible, do your workouts where you'll be doing your race. If not, no big deal. Don't do the workouts back to back; take plenty of time in between.

Swim: Very short 10-minute swim. Just get loose.

Bike: 10- to 30-minute easy ride. Run through each of the gears on the bike and be sure the tire pressure is just right.

Run: 10- to 15-minute easy run.

Day 7 *Race day!*

Training Plan for a Sprint Triathlon

Now that you've read the day-by-day description of what is on the plan, you can better use the chart on the following page to get a quick overview of what you're doing on any given day/week/month. You can make a copy of the program and hang it on your fridge so the family knows what you're up to.

The Least You Need to Know

- ◆ Don't let TRI control your life; make it work with your schedule.
- ◆ Understand the specific drills you'll be performing *before* you start your workout.
- ◆ Following this day-by-day sprint training program will get you prepared for your sprint race.

WEEK	Sport	M	T	W	T	F	S	S	Total (min.)	Totals
1	Swim	20			25		O 15		60	1 hr. 0 min.
	Bike			45			45		90	1 hr. 30 min.
	Run		30				T 10	37	77	1 hr. 17 min.
	Other			W 30			S 30	W 30	90	1 hr. 30 min.
2	Swim	25			25		O 15		65	1 hr. 5 min.
	Bike			45			55		100	1 hr. 40 min.
	Run		35	0			T 10	40	85	1 hr. 25 min.
	Other			W 30			S 30	W 30	90	1 hr. 30 min.
3	Swim	25			30		O 15		70	1 hr. 10 min.
	Bike			45			65		110	1 hr. 50 min.
	Run		35				T 10	45	90	1 hr. 30 min.
	Other			W 30			S 30	W 30	90	1 hr. 30 min.
4 Recover	Swim	20		0	25				45	0 hr. 45 min.
	Bike			35			50		85	1 hr. 25 min.
	Run		30	0			T 10	35	75	1 hr. 15 min.
	Other			W 30			S 30	W 30	90	1 hr. 30 min.
5	Swim	30		0	35		O 12		77	1 hr. 17 min.
	Bike	T 10		40			70		120	2 hr. 0 min.
	Run		35	0			T 15	45	95	1 hr. 35 min.
	Other			W 30			S 30	W 30	90	1 hr. 30 min.
6	Swim	35			40		10		85	1 hr. 25 min.
	Bike			50			82		132	2 hr. 12 min.
	Run		35	OT 10			T 15	50	110	1 hr. 50 min.
	Other			W 30			S 30	W 30	90	1 hr. 30 min.
7	Swim	40			40		O 15		95	1 hr. 35 min.
	Bike			55			90		145	2 hr. 25 min.
	Run		35				T 15	55	105	1 hr. 45 min.
	Other			W 30			S 30	W 30	90	1 hr. 30 min.
8 Recover	Swim	30			30		O 15		75	1 hr. 15 min.
	Bike			50			60		110	1 hr. 50 min.
	Run		30				T 10	40	80	1 hr. 20 min.
	Other						S 30		30	0 hr. 30 min.
9	Swim	40			40		O 15		95	1 hr. 35 min.
	Bike			50			75		125	2 hr. 5 min.
	Run		35				T 10	60	105	1 hr. 45 min.
	Other			W 30			S 30	W 30	90	1 hr. 30 min.
10	Swim	40			40		O 15		95	1 hr. 35 min.
	Bike	T 10		45			65		120	2 hr. 0 min.
	Run		35				T 10	50	95	1 hr. 35 min.
	Other			W 30			S 30	W 30	90	1 hr. 30 min.
11 Taper	Swim	35			30		O 20		85	1 hr. 25 min.
	Bike			45			55		100	1 hr. 40 min.
	Run		30				T 10	40	80	1 hr. 20 min.
	Other						S 30		30	0 hr. 30 min.
12 Race	Swim	30			30		10		70	1 hr. 10 min.
	Bike			45			30		75	1 hr. 15 min.
	Run		25		20		15		60	1 hr. 0 min.
	Other						S 30		30	0 hr. 30 min.

O = optional
T = transition
W = weights
S = stretch

Chapter 14

Beyond the Sprint

In This Chapter

- ◆ Workout charts and tips on how to use them
- ◆ Master workout training plans for super-sprint, Olympic, half-Ironman, and Ironman distance races
- ◆ Specific workouts for each TRI-sport in each distance training program

If you've decided to do a race other than a sprint, and you've been able to find one that works with your schedule and budget, this is the chapter for you. Although we won't get into as much detail as we did with the sprint distance program in Chapter 13, we still do give you all the information you need to feel confident and succeed in your training and race. That said, if you skipped it because you thought it wouldn't apply to you, go back and check it out. Although the exact workouts won't match your program, the philosophy and methodology are the same.

In this chapter, along with the charts that showcase the number of minutes you might want to spend on each sport each day, we give you specific workouts you can do in each sport, with different options for all three sports.

You typically want to have one speed workout and one longer workout in each sport per week (the essence of TRI training). Other workouts are peppered into the schedule, but they generally won't be long or hard. There is no exact science to a training program, but one long workout and one speed workout per sport is a generally accepted practice. Listen to your body and intuition (and your loved ones), and customize as necessary.

Gravel Ahead _____

Keep in mind that speed is a relative thing. Many beginners might not get fully into "speed workouts" when just starting out. However, you can apply speed in your program without getting injured. Just take it easy and gradually. If you typically run a mile at the track in 11 minutes, perhaps your speed day interval would be a clip at a 10- or 10.5-minute pace.

Cracking the Code

The super-sprint, Olympic, half-Ironman, and Ironman schedules all include an overview chart that suggests the amount of time you should spend on each sport each day. For any nonspeed workouts for biking and running, you only need to check out the suggested minutes of training and go out for a nice and easy workout at that pace. If you see "30" in the running row of a given day, it simply means lace up your shoes and run (or run/walk) for about 30 minutes. The same goes for the bike. Generally speaking, keep your heart rate in zones 1 and 2 for these standard workouts.

Swim Enlightenment

The majority of swims (those not marked as "optional") are set up as interval workouts. Speed and number of laps vary, but you have several workout options for your time in the water. Even the "long" swims are set up as interval sets to keep you focused and keep your mind active while you're in sensory depravation. If you try to just swim for a designated number of minutes instead of doing a specific workout, it might drive you batty. That said, if swimming for a specific number of minutes works best for you, adjust as necessary.

On any nonoptional day of swimming, you can choose one of the workouts from the specific interval workouts for your race distance. Because most of the interval workouts have varying total distances, the time almost never exactly matches what's in your overall schedule. Adjust the workout as necessary, and keep in mind that swimming is the one sport of TRI where pushing a little harder or going a little longer than planned won't negatively impact your program.

If you choose to do a specific workout and you reach the designated time before you complete the workout, you can cut yourself off at that point, after you do your cool-down set. If you go over the designated time to complete the workout, don't worry about it. Additionally, we didn't put a unit of measure on the distances in the specific interval workouts, as some pools are measured in meters and some in yards. These two distances are similar, so you can just use the numbers in the workout descriptions and assume we meant the unit by which your pool is measured.

Coaches' Corner
At most pools, the length of a lap lane is either 25 meters or 25 yards. If the distance across your pool is different, don't panic! The most important aspect of the workout is the amount of time you spend swimming. Adjust the workouts as necessary to fit your pool's length. If possible, try to find a pool that's at least 20 meters or 20 yards long so you have enough room to stretch your form out.

Bike and Run 411

As a rule of thumb, each sport should have one "long" workout and one speed workout each week. If you're just starting out and don't feel comfortable with speed workouts, feel free to postpone them until you're ready. If you are ready, however, insert a tempo, fartlek, or interval workout each week. When adding speed to the schedule, try to follow these two guidelines:

1. Do not schedule a speed workout if there is already a speed workout or long workout for bike or run that day.

2. Try to stick primarily to fartleks for speed workouts during recovery weeks.

We spoke about tempo workouts and fartleks in Chapter 7. If you only skimmed over it or have never done these types of workouts, you might want to revisit Chapter 7. Although there are no "fartlek bike workouts," we do schedule tempo rides. Both tempo workouts and fartleks are done with a warm-up, the main workout, and then the cool-down.

Because interval workouts are more than just upping your pace for a specific amount of time, we give you several workout options to choose from.

As you get closer to race day, when selecting interval workouts, try to choose those that have fewer sets and longer repetitions/durations.

Remember, most of the specific bike workouts are best accomplished on an indoor trainer. If you choose to attempt them outdoors, use common sense and stay safe.

Training Tips _____

As with everything we suggest in this book, feel free to tweak the workouts as needed to fit your needs and abilities. We offer a road map to get from A to B, but don't be afraid to take a slight detour when you need to.

The Heart of It All

Because we're not writing out day-by-day instructions for each of these nonsprint training programs, we cannot give super-specific recommendations on heart rate zones. We're confident you'll be able to handle this part of the program on your own. In Chapter 4, we went into some in-depth discussion about the different phases of training and where your heart rate should be during hard workouts in those phases. (Turn back there if you need a refresher.)

We've labeled the weeks by phase in the daily workout charts in each program. Although not shown in the daily charts, remember that during the Prep phase, you should try to remain primarily in zone 1 (Z1). For the other phases, long workouts should be done in Z1 and Z2. Harder/speed workouts should follow these general guidelines:

Gravel Ahead

Try to follow the heart rate zone recommendations. Pushing yourself into higher zones on a regular basis very early in the program could lead to burnout.

Phase	Zone(s)
Base (lightest shade on chart)	primarily Z1 and Z2 (some Z3 okay)
Build (medium shade on chart)	primarily Z2 and Z3 (some Z4 okay)
Peak (darkest shade on chart)	primarily Z3 and Z4

Level of Exertion Recap

Description	Zone	Percent of Max Heart Rate	RPE
Active recovery	1	55 to 65	12 to 13
Endurance	2	65 to 75	13 to 15
Resistance	3	75 to 85	15 to 16
Threshold	4	85 to 90	16 to 18

Whether you're wearing a heart rate monitor or using your rate of perceived exertion, the level at which you should be pushing yourself during hard/speed workouts should correspond with these principles.

In addition to the heart rate adjustments that should occur between the phases, try to make an adjustment with regards to your interval workouts. As you get closer to your race, try to choose workouts with longer intervals. You'll benefit from the longer duration workouts because they'll really simulate race conditions.

Take It Up a Notch

The more advanced triathletes can adjust workouts in a couple different ways. The easiest way is to simply add 5 to 10 percent to the duration shown in the charts. Additionally, during speed workouts, you might want to add one or two extra reps to the sets. The key is to balance between time and task. In other words, if you finish what's on the programs 10 minutes earlier than the target duration, adjust your workout accordingly.

You could also incorporate a couple workouts from the training program one step longer than your program (if you're training for an Olympic, incorporate a couple half-Ironman workouts). If you decide to incorporate some workouts from a training program for a longer race, do that primarily in the base or build phase. When you get into the peak phase, you'll want to get back to the shorter workouts of your own program in specific preparation for your race.

Strong and Limber

We've put two suggested sessions of weight lifting and one suggested session of stretching in most weeks of each training plan. As discussed in Chapter 12, adjust the placement of these sessions as necessary. Follow your common sense or your doctor's orders, or get some personal advice from a trainer/mentor. (See Chapter 10 for further details on weight training and flexibility.)

Coaches' Corner
When we say you should feel free to adjust these programs/workouts as your body tells you, we really mean it. Steve likes to divide his long workouts for the bike and run with a few days of standard training in between. Colin prefers to utilize the weekends to get these long sessions done, so following the TRI order, he does his long bike rides on Saturdays and his long runs on Sundays. Both methods work. The most important thing is that your program works for *you*.

One Last Thing

Although Day 6 and Day 7 are assumed to be the weekend in our training charts, don't think you have to be locked into those days. Adjust the schedule so that you can train and still have time for all the other important things in your life!

Super-Sprint

WEEK	Sport	M	T	W	T	F	S	S	Total (min.)	Totals
1	Swim	10			12		O 10		32	0 hr. 32 min.
	Bike			20			25		45	0 hr. 45 min.
	Run				15		T 10	20	45	0 hr. 45 min.
	Other			W 30			S 30	W 30	90	1 hr. 30 min.
2	Swim	12			14		O 10		36	0 hr. 36 min.
	Bike			20			30		50	0 hr. 50 min.
	Run				17		T 10	23	50	0 hr. 50 min.
	Other			W 30			S 30	W 30	90	1 hr. 30 min.
3	Swim	16			15		O 10		41	0 hr. 41 min.
	Bike	T 10		22			35		67	1 hr. 7 min.
	Run				18		T 10	27	55	0 hr. 55 min.
	Other			W 30			S 30	W 30	90	1 hr. 30 min.
4 Recover	Swim	15			14				29	0 hr. 29 min.
	Bike			20			25		45	0 hr. 45 min.
	Run				15		T 10	20	45	0 hr. 45 min.
	Other			W 30			S 30	W 30	90	1 hr. 30 min.
5	Swim	18			18		O 11		47	0 hr. 47 min.
	Bike			33			40		73	1 hr. 13 min.
	Run				20		T 10	31	61	1 hr. 1 min.
	Other			W 30			S 30	W 30	90	1 hr. 30 min.
6	Swim	18			25		O 10		53	0 hr. 53 min.
	Bike	T 10		35			45		90	1 hr. 30 min.
	Run				17		T 10	40	67	1 hr. 7 min.
	Other			W 30			S 30	W 30	90	1 hr. 30 min.
7 Taper	Swim	20			20		O 10		50	0 hr. 50 min.
	Bike			35			35		70	1 hr. 10 min.
	Run				22		T 10	30	62	1 hr. 2 min.
	Other			W 30			S 30	W 30	90	1 hr. 30 min.
8 Race	Swim	15			15		10		40	0 hr. 40 min.
	Bike			30			15		45	0 hr. 45 min.
	Run				20		10		30	0 hr. 30 min.
	Other						S 30		30	0 hr. 30 min.

O = optional
T = transition
W = weights
S = stretch

Swim Workouts

HARD	Reps		Dist.	Inten.	Rest
Warm-up	3	x	50		15
Set	1	x	100		30
	10	x	25	+	10
	1	x	100		30
Cool-down	3	x	50		15

	Reps		Dist.	Inten.	Rest
Warm-up	4	x	25		15
Set	6	x	50		15
	6	x	25	+	10
Cool-down	2	x	50		20

	Reps		Dist.	Inten.	Rest
Warm-up	3	x	50		15
Set	6	x	75		10
Cool-down	4	x	25		15

LONG	Reps		Dist.	Inten.	Rest
Warm-up	3	x	50		15
Set	3	x	200		35
Cool-down	2	x	50		15

	Reps		Dist.	Inten.	Rest
Warm-up	4	x	50		15
Set	2	x	300		40
Cool-down	2	x	100		15

	Reps		Dist.	Inten.	Rest
Warm-up	3	x	50		15
Set	5	x	100		20
Cool-down	6	x	25		15

Bike Workouts

Intervals	Reps		Time	Rest	Inten.	Spec.
Warm-up	1	x	10			
Set	4	x	1	2		
Cool-down	1	x	7			

Intervals	Reps		Time	Rest	Inten.	Spec.
Warm-up	1	x	10			
Set	4	x	2	1		
Cool-down	1	x	7			

Intervals	Reps		Time	Rest	Inten.	Spec.
Warm-up	1	x	10			
Set	4	x	0.5	1		SLD
	2	x	1	1	+	BGD
	2	x	1	1		SGD
Cool-down	1	x	7			

Intervals	Reps		Time	Rest	Inten.	Spec.
Warm-up	1	x	10			
Set	2	x	5	2		
Cool-down	1	x	7			

Intervals	Reps		Time	Rest	Inten.	Spec.
Warm-up	1	x	10			
Set	8	x	1	1		
Cool-down	1	x	7			

Intervals	Reps		Time	Rest	Inten.	Spec.
Warm-up	1	x	10			
Set	12	x	1			SLD
Cool-down	1	x	7			

Run Workouts

Intervals	Reps		Time	Rest	Inten.
Warm-up	1	x	7		
Set	5	x	0.5	0.5	
Cool-down	1	x	7		

Intervals	Reps		Time	Rest	Inten.
Warm-up	1	x	7		
Set	1	x	2	1	
	2	x	1	0.5	+
Cool-down	1	x	7		

Intervals	Reps		Time	Rest	Inten.
Warm-up	1	x	10		
Set	5	x	1	1	
Cool-down	1	x	5		

Olympic

WEEK	Sport	M	T	W	T	F	S	S	Total (min.)	Totals
1	Swim	25			25		O 10		60	1 hr. 0 min.
	Bike			35			65		100	1 hr. 40 min.
	Run		25				T 15	40	80	1 hr. 20 min.
	Other			W 30			S 30	W 30	90	1 hr. 30 min.
2	Swim	27			30		O 10		67	1 hr. 7 min.
	Bike			40			70		110	1 hr. 50 min.
	Run		20	T 10			T 15	43	88	1 hr. 28 min.
	Other			W 30			S 30	W 30	90	1 hr. 30 min.
3	Swim	30			35		O 10		75	1 hr. 15 min.
	Bike			45			75		120	2 hr. 0 min.
	Run		25	T 10			T 15	47	97	1 hr. 37 min.
	Other			W 30			S 30	W 30	90	1 hr. 30 min.
4 Recover	Swim	25			30				55	0 hr. 55 min.
	Bike			30			60		90	1 hr. 30 min.
	Run		25				T 10	35	70	1 hr. 10 min.
	Other			W 30			S 30	W 30	90	1 hr. 30 min.
5	Swim	35			35		O 12		82	1 hr. 22 min.
	Bike			45			87		132	2 hr. 12 min.
	Run		30	T 10			T 15	53	108	1 hr. 48 min.
	Other			W 30			S 30	W 30	90	1 hr. 30 min.
6	Swim	35			40		O 15		90	1 hr. 30 min.
	Bike			50			95		145	2 hr. 25 min.
	Run		35	T 10			T 17	56	118	1 hr. 58 min.
	Other			W 30			S 30	W 30	90	1 hr. 30 min.
7	Swim	40			45		O 15		100	1 hr. 40 min.
	Bike	T 15		40			105		160	2 hr. 40 min.
	Run		36	T 10			T 18	66	130	2 hr. 10 min.
	Other			W 30			S 30	W 30	90	1 hr. 30 min.

continues

continued

WEEK	Sport	M	T	W	T	F	S	S	Total (min.)	Totals
8 Recover	Swim	30		0	36				66	1 hr. 6 min.
	Bike			45			80		125	2 hr. 5 min.
	Run		27	7			T 10	49	93	1 hr. 33 min.
	Other			W 30			S 30	W 30	90	1 hr. 30 min.
9	Swim	45			50		15		110	1 hr. 50 min.
	Bike			50			125		175	2 hr. 55 min.
	Run		45	T 10			T 15	73	143	2 hr. 23 min.
	Other			W 30			S 30	W 30	90	1 hr. 30 min.
10	Swim	50			57		15		122	2 hr. 1 min.
	Bike			60			135		195	3 hr. 15 min.
	Run		50	T 10			T 15	82	157	2 hr. 37 min.
	Other			W 30			S 30	W 30	90	1 hr. 30 min.
11	Swim	55			60		O 20		135	2 hr. 15 min.
	Bike			65			150		215	3 hr. 35 min.
	Run		53	T 10			T 20	90	173	2 hr. 53 min.
	Other			W 30			S 30	W 30	90	1 hr. 30 min.
12 Recover	Swim	40			50		O 15		105	1 hr. 45 min.
	Bike			60			105		165	2 hr. 45 min.
	Run		40				T 15	70	125	2 hr. 5 min.
	Other						S 30		30	0 hr. 30 min.
13	Swim	50			60		O 15		125	2 hr. 5 min.
	Bike	T 20		60			130		210	3 hr. 30 min.
	Run		55				T 20	80	155	2 hr. 35 min.
	Other			W 30			S 30	W 30	90	1 hr. 30 min.
14	Swim	45			60		O 15		120	2 hr. 0 min.
	Bike	T 10		55			115		180	3 hr. 0 min.
	Run		55				T 20	70	145	2 hr. 25 min.
	Other			W 30			S 30	W 30	90	1 hr. 30 min.
15 Taper	Swim	35			35		O 20		90	1 hr. 30 min.
	Bike			55			80		135	2 hr. 15 min.
	Run		40				T 15	45	100	1 hr. 40 min.
	Other						S 30		30	0 hr. 30 min.
16 Race	Swim	30			30		10		70	1 hr. 10 min.
	Bike			60			30		90	1 hr. 30 min.
	Run		30		20		15		65	1 hr. 5 min.
	Other			S 30					30	0 hr. 30 min.

O = optional
T = transition
W = weights
S = stretch

Swim Workouts

HARD	Reps		Dist.	Inten.	Rest
Warm-up	6	x	50		15
Set	1	x	250		30
	25	x	25	+	10
	2	x	250		30
Cool-down	3	x	100		15

	Reps		Dist.	Inten.	Rest
Warm-up	2	x	150		15
Set	10	x	100	+	15
	10	x	50	++	10
Cool-down	4	x	100		20

	Reps		Dist.	Inten.	Rest
Warm-up	5	x	100		15
Set	9	x	100		15
	9	x	50	+	10
	9	x	25	++	5
Cool-down	1	x	300		15

LONG	Reps		Dist.	Inten.	Rest
Warm-up	8	x	50		15
Set	3	x	100	+	15
	2	x	200		25
	3	x	100	+	15
	2	x	200		25
	3	x	100	+	15
	2	x	200		25
Cool-down	4	x	100		15

	Reps		Dist.	Inten.	Rest
Warm-up	4	x	100		15
Set	6	x	50	++	10
	8	x	100	+	15
	4	x	200		20
Cool-Down	4	x	150		15

	Reps		Dist.	Inten.	Rest
Warm-up	3	x	150		5
Set	4	x	500		60
Cool-down	4	x	100		10

Bike Workouts

Intervals	Reps		Time	Rest	Inten.	Spec.
Warm-up	1	x	10			
Set	8	x	1	2		
Cool-down	1	x	10			

Intervals	Reps		Time	Rest	Inten.	Spec.
Warm-up	1	x	15			
Set	7	x	2	1	+	Hard
	3	x	1	1		BGD
	3	x	1	1		SGD
Cool-down	1	x	10			

Intervals	Reps		Time	Rest	Inten.	Spec.
Warm-up	1	x	15			
Set	10	x	1	0		SLD
	5	x	1	1	+	BGD
	5	x	1	1	+	SGD
Cool-down	1	x	10			

Intervals	Reps		Time	Rest	Inten.	Spec.
Warm-up	1	x	15			
Set	5	x	5	2		
Cool-down	1	x	10			

Intervals	Reps		Time	Rest	Inten.	Spec.
Warm-up	1	x	15			
Set	5	x	5	2		
Cool-down	1	x	10			

Intervals	Reps		Time	Rest	Inten.	Spec.
Warm-up	1	x	15			
Set	5	x	1	1	+	
	5	x	1	0	+	
	10	x	0.5	0		
Cool-down	1	x	15			

Intervals	Reps		Time	Rest	Inten.	Spec.
Warm-up	1	x	15			
Set	1	x	5	1		Hard
	12	x	1	0		SLD
	1	x	5	1	+	Hard
Cool-down	1	x	10			

Intervals	Reps		Time	Rest	Inten.	Spec.
Warm-up	1	x	15			
Set	5	x	1	1	+	
	5	x	1	0	+	
	10	x	0.5	0		
Cool-down	1	x	15			

Run Workouts

Intervals	Reps		Time	Rest	Inten.
Warm-up	1	x	15		
Set	4	x	1	1	
	4	x	2	1	+
Cool-down	1	x	10		

Intervals	Reps		Time	Rest	Inten.
Warm-up	1	x	15		
Set	3	x	2	0.5	+
	1	x	6	4	
	2	x	3	2	++
Cool-down	1	x	15		

Intervals	Reps		Time	Rest	Inten.
Warm-up	1	x	15		
Set	3	x	2	2	
Cool-down	1	x	10		

Intervals	Reps		Time	Rest	Inten.
Warm-up	1	x	20		
Set	3	x	5	2	
Cool-down	1	x	15		

Half-Ironman

WEEK	Sport	M	T	W	T	F	S	S	Total (min.)	Totals		
1	Swim	28		25	35		20		108	1 hr.	48	min.
	Bike	35		35			65		135	2 hr.	15	min.
	Run		25 T	10	35	T	15	40	125	2 hr.	5	min.
	Other				W 30		S 30	W 30	90	1 hr.	30	min.
2	Swim	32		30	40		20		122	2 hr.	1	min.
	Bike	35		35			80		150	2 hr.	30	min.
	Run		30 T	10	35	T	15	45	135	2 hr.	15	min.
	Other				W 30		S 30	W 30	90	1 hr.	30	min.
3	Swim	35		35	45		O 20		135	2 hr.	15	min.
	Bike	T 15	30	30			90		165	2 hr.	45	min.
	Run		35 T	10	35	T	15	50	145	2 hr.	25	min.
	Other				W 30		S 30	W 30	90	1 hr.	30	min.
4 Recover	Swim	35		35	30				100	1 hr.	40	min.
	Bike	30		35			60		125	2 hr.	5	min.
	Run		25		35	T	10	35	105	1 hr.	45	min.
	Other				W 30		S 30	W 30	90	1 hr.	30	min.
5	Swim	40		35	45		25		145	2 hr.	25	min.
	Bike	35		45			100		180	3 hr.	0	min.
	Run		35 T	15	35	T	20	55	160	2 hr.	40	min.
	Other				W 30		S 30	W 30	90	1 hr.	30	min.
6	Swim	45		40	40		30		155	2 hr.	35	min.
	Bike	40		45			115		200	3 hr.	20	min.
	Run		40 T	15	40	T	20	60	175	2 hr.	55	min.
	Other				W 30		S 30	W 30	90	1 hr.	30	min.

continues

continued

WEEK	Sport	M	T	W	T	F	S	S	Total (min.)	Totals
7	Swim	50		40	45		O 30		165	2 hr. 45 min.
	Bike	T 15	30	50			125		220	3 hr. 40 min.
	Run		45	T 15	40		T 20	65	185	3 hr. 5 min.
	Other				W 30		S 30	W 30	90	1 hr. 30 min.
8 Recover	Swim	45		40	30				115	1 hr. 55 min.
	Bike	40		45			75		160	2 hr. 40 min.
	Run		30	T 15	30		T 10	50	135	2 hr. 15 min.
	Other				W 30		S 30	W 30	90	1 hr. 30 min.
9	Swim	55		45	50		30		180	3 hr. 0 min.
	Bike	45		55			140		240	4 hr. 0 min.
	Run		45	T 15	45		T 20	75	200	3 hr. 20 min.
	Other				W 30		S 30	W 30	90	1 hr. 30 min.
10	Swim	60		50	60		30		200	3 hr. 20 min.
	Bike	50		60			155		265	4 hr. 25 min.
	Run		50	T 15	45		T 20	85	215	3 hr. 35 min.
	Other				W 30		S 30	W 30	90	1 hr. 30 min.
11	Swim	65		55	65		O 30		215	3 hr. 35 min.
	Bike	55		70			170		295	4 hr. 55 min.
	Run		55	T 15	45		T 25	90	230	3 hr. 50 min.
	Other				W 30		S 30	W 30	90	1 hr. 30 min.
12 Recover	Swim	65		40	65		O 25		195	3 hr. 15 min.
	Bike	45		60			115		220	3 hr. 40 min.
	Run		40	T 10	40		T 15	65	170	2 hr. 50 min.
	Other				W 30		S 30		60	1 hr. 0 min.
13	Swim	70		60	75		O 30		235	3 hr. 55 min.
	Bike	60		75			190		325	5 hr. 25 min.
	Run		65	T 15	50		T 25	95	250	4 hr. 10 min.
	Other				W 30		S 30	W 30	90	1 hr. 30 min.
14	Swim	75		60	75		O 30		240	4 hr. 0 min.
	Bike	60		80			215		355	5 hr. 55 min.
	Run		70	T 15	45		T 25	105	260	4 hr. 20 min.
	Other				W 30		S 30	W 30	90	1 hr. 30 min.
15	Swim	75		65	75		O 30		245	4 hr. 5 min.
	Bike	60		85			240		385	6 hr. 25 min.
	Run		75	T 15	45		T 25	120	280	4 hr. 40 min.
	Other				W 30		S 30	W 30	90	1 hr. 30 min.
16 Recover	Swim	65		40	60		O 25		190	3 hr. 10 min.
	Bike	45		60			165		270	4 hr. 30 min.
	Run		60	T 10	35		T 15	85	205	3 hr. 25 min.
	Other				W 30		S 30		60	1 hr. 0 min.
17	Swim	65		60	65		O 25		215	3 hr. 35 min.
	Bike	T 20	50	70			180		320	5 hr. 20 min.
	Run		75	T 10	40		T 25	105	255	4 hr. 15 min.
	Other				W 30		S 30	W 30	90	1 hr. 30 min.
18	Swim	45		60	65		O 25		195	3 hr. 15 min.
	Bike	70		70			150		290	4 hr. 50 min.
	Run		70	T 10	40		T 25	90	235	3 hr. 55 min.
	Other				W 30		S 30	W 30	90	1 hr. 30 min.
19 Taper	Swim	45		60	65		O 25		195	3 hr. 15 min.
	Bike	65		70			150		285	4 hr. 45 min.
	Run		70	T 10	40		T 25	75	220	3 hr. 40 min.
	Other				W 30		S 30	W 30	90	1 hr. 30 min.
20 Race	Swim	55		55	45		10		165	2 hr. 45 min.
	Bike	55		75			30		160	2 hr. 40 min.
	Run		65	T 10	40		15		130	2 hr. 10 min.
	Other			S 30					30	0 hr. 30 min.

O = optional
T = transition
W = weights
S = stretch

Swim Workouts

HARD	Reps		Dist.	Inten.	Rest
Warm-up	5	x	100		15
Set	1	x	200		30
	15	x	100	+	25
	1	x	200		30
Cool-down	2	x	200		15

	Reps		Dist.	Inten.	Rest
Warm-up	4	x	150		15
Set	8	x	100		15
	20	x	50	+	10
Cool-down	4	x	100		20

	Reps		Dist.	Inten.	Rest
Warm-up	5	x	100		15
Set	9	x	100		15
	9	x	50	+	10
	9	x	25	++	5
Cool-down	1	x	300		15

LONG	Reps		Dist.	Inten.	Rest
Warm-up	4	x	100		15
Set	3	x	300		30
	2	x	100	+	15
	3	x	300		30
Cool-down	4	x	150		15

	Reps		Dist.	Inten.	Rest
Warm-up	8	x	50		15
Set	2	x	100	+	15
	4	x	200		25
	2	x	100	+	15
	4	x	200		25
Cool-down	5	x	100		15

	Reps		Dist.	Inten.	Rest
Warm-up	6	x	75		5
Set	5	x	500		60
Cool-down	4	x	100		10

Bike Workouts

Intervals	Reps		Time	Rest	Inten.	Spec.
Warm-up	1	x	15			
Set	10	x	2	3	Desc.	
Cool-down	1	x	10			

Intervals	Reps		Time	Rest	Inten.	Spec.
Warm-up	1	x	15			
Set	5	x	2	1	+	Hard
	3	x	2	1		BGD
	5	x	2	1		SGD
Cool-down	1	x	10			

Intervals	Reps		Time	Rest	Inten.	Spec.
Warm-up	1	x	15			
Set	6	x	1	0		SLD
	5	x	1	1	+	BGD
	6	x	1	0		SLD
	5	x	1	1	+	SGD
	6	x	1	0	+	SLD
Cool-down	1	x	10			

Intervals	Reps		Time	Rest	Inten.	Spec.
Warm-up	1	x	15			
Set	5	x	5	3	+	
Cool-down	1	x	10			

Intervals	Reps		Time	Rest	Inten.	Spec.
Warm-up	1	x	15			
Set	10	x	2	1		BGD
	10	x	1	0	+	
	20	x	0.5	0		SLD
Cool-down	1	x	15			

Intervals	Reps		Time	Rest	Inten.	Spec.
Warm-up	1	x	15			
Set	1	x	7	1		Hard
	20	x	1	0		SLD
	1	x	7	1		Hard
Cool-down	1	x	10			

Run Workouts

Intervals	Reps		Time	Rest	Inten.
Warm-up	1	x	15		
Set	3	x	3	2	
	5	x	2	2	+
Cool-down	1	x	10		

Intervals	Reps		Time	Rest	Inten.
Warm-up	1	x	15		
Set	6	x	3	2	
Cool-down	1	x	10		

Intervals	Reps		Time	Rest	Inten.
Warm-up	1	x	20		
Set	3	x	2	1	+
	2	x	4	2	
	1	x	8	0	
Cool-down	1	x	15		

Intervals	Reps		Time	Rest	Inten.
Warm-up	1	x	20		
Set	4	x	5	3	
Cool-down	1	x	15		

Ironman

WEEK	Sport	M	T	W	T	F	S	S	Total (min.)	Totals
1	Swim	45		45	45				135	2 hr. 15 min.
	Bike	60		60			97		217	3 hr. 37 min.
	Run		35		40		T 15	50	140	2 hr. 20 min.
	Other			W 30			S 30	W 30	90	1 hr. 30 min.
2	Swim	55		35	45		20		155	2 hr. 35 min.
	Bike	60		60			107		227	3 hr. 47 min.
	Run		40		43		T 15	55	153	2 hr. 33 min.
	Other			W 30			S 30	W 30	90	1 hr. 30 min.
3	Swim	65		35	55		O 20		175	2 hr. 55 min.
	Bike	T 15	50	60			119		244	4 hr. 4 min.
	Run		45	10	40		T 14	60	169	2 hr. 49 min.
	Other			W 30			S 30	W 30	90	1 hr. 30 min.
4 Recover	Swim	60		30	55				145	2 hr. 25 min.
	Bike	50		45			89		184	3 hr. 4 min.
	Run		35	10	30		T 10	45	130	2 hr. 10 min.
	Other			W 30			S 30	W 30	90	1 hr. 30 min.
5	Swim	75		30	75		20		200	3 hr. 20 min.
	Bike	75		60			132		267	4 hr. 27 min.
	Run		50	T 10	45		T 15	65	185	3 hr. 5 min.
	Other			W 30			S 30	W 30	90	1 hr. 30 min.
6	Swim	80		45	75		20		220	3 hr. 40 min.
	Bike	75		70			147		292	4 hr. 52 min.
	Run		55	T 10	45		T 15	75	200	3 hr. 20 min.
	Other			W 30			S 30	W 30	90	1 hr. 30 min.
7	Swim	90		45	90		O 20		245	4 hr. 5 min.
	Bike	T 20	70	70			164		324	5 hr. 24 min.
	Run		60	10	45		T 14	80	209	3 hr. 29 min.
	Other			W 30			S 30	W 30	90	1 hr. 30 min.
8 Recover	Swim	75		35	75		O 15		200	3 hr. 20 min.
	Bike	60		55			123		238	3 hr. 58 min.
	Run		40	10	35		T 10	60	155	2 hr. 35 min.
	Other			W 30			S 30	W 30	90	1 hr. 30 min.
9	Swim	90		55	90		30		265	4 hr. 25 min.
	Bike	90		80			182		352	5 hr. 52 min.
	Run		60	T 10	50		T 15	90	225	3 hr. 45 min.
	Other			W 30			S 30	W 30	90	1 hr. 30 min.
10	Swim	90		65	90		30		275	4 hr. 35 min.
	Bike	90		80			202		372	6 hr. 12 min.
	Run		65	T 10	50		T 15	90	230	3 hr. 50 min.
	Other			W 30			S 30	W 30	90	1 hr. 30 min.
11	Swim	90		75	90		30		285	4 hr. 45 min.
	Bike	T 30	70	80			224		404	6 hr. 44 min.
	Run		70	T 10	50		T 14	95	239	3 hr. 59 min.
	Other			W 30			S 30	W 30	90	1 hr. 30 min.
12 Recover	Swim	75		55	70		O 25		225	3 hr. 45 min.
	Bike	60		60			168		288	4 hr. 48 min.
	Run		50	10	40		T 10	60	170	2 hr. 50 min.
	Other			W 30			S 30	W 30	90	1 hr. 30 min.
13	Swim	90		75	90		35		290	4 hr. 50 min.
	Bike	90		90			249		429	7 hr. 9 min.
	Run		75	T 10	55		T 15	105	260	4 hr. 20 min.
	Other			W 30			S 30	W 30	90	1 hr. 30 min.
14	Swim	90		75	90		40		295	4 hr. 55 min.
	Bike	90		90			277		457	7 hr. 37 min.
	Run		75	T 10	60		T 15	120	280	4 hr. 40 min.
	Other			W 30			S 30	W 30	90	1 hr. 30 min.
15	Swim	90		75	90		45		300	5 hr. 0 min.
	Bike	T 45	55	90			308		498	8 hr. 18 min.
	Run		75	15	60		T 25	130	305	5 hr. 5 min.
	Other			W 30			S 30	W 30	90	1 hr. 30 min.

WEEK	Sport	M	T	W	T	F	S	S	Total (min.)	Totals
16 Recover	Swim	75		55	75		O 20		225	3 hr. 45 min.
	Bike	60		50			231		341	5 hr. 41 min.
	Run		56	10	45		T 15	98	224	3 hr. 44 min.
	Other			W 30			S 30	W 30	90	1 hr. 30 min.
17	Swim	90		80	90		45		305	5 hr. 5 min.
	Bike	90		90			342		522	8 hr. 42 min.
	Run		75 T	15	65		45	135	335	5 hr. 35 min.
	Other			W 30			S 30	W 30	90	1 hr. 30 min.
18	Swim	90		80	90		45		305	5 hr. 5 min.
	Bike	90		90			380		560	9 hr. 20 min.
	Run		75 T	15	75		30	150	345	5 hr. 45 min.
	Other			W 30			S 30	W 30	90	1 hr. 30 min.
19	Swim	90		80	90		O 45		305	5 hr. 5 min.
	Bike	T 45	55	90			420		610	10 hr. 10 min.
	Run		75 T	15	75		40	120	325	5 hr. 25 min.
	Other			W 30			S 30	W 30	90	1 hr. 30 min.
20 Recover	Swim	55		55	45		10		165	2 hr. 45 min.
	Bike	55		75			30	60	220	3 hr. 40 min.
	Run		65 T	10	40		15		130	2 hr. 10 min.
	Other			S 30					30	0 hr. 30 min.
21	Swim	75		60	75		O 30		240	4 hr. 0 min.
	Bike	T 20	50	70			180		320	5 hr. 20 min.
	Run		75 T	10	40		25	105	255	4 hr. 15 min.
	Other			S 30					30	0 hr. 30 min.
22	Swim	75		60	75		O 30		240	4 hr. 0 min.
	Bike	70		70			150		290	4 hr. 50 min.
	Run		70 T	10	40		25	90	235	3 hr. 55 min.
	Other			S 30					30	0 hr. 30 min.
23 Taper	Swim	75		60	75		O 30		240	4 hr. 0 min.
	Bike	65		70			120		255	4 hr. 15 min.
	Run		70 T	10	40		25	75	220	3 hr. 40 min.
	Other			S 30					30	0 hr. 30 min.
24 Race	Swim	60		45	30		10		145	2 hr. 25 min.
	Bike	60		45			30		135	2 hr. 15 min.
	Run		40 T	10	30		15		95	1 hr. 35 min.
	Other			S 30					30	0 hr. 30 min.

O = optional
T = transition
W = weights
S = stretch

Swim Workouts

HARD	Reps		Dist.	Inten.	Rest
Warm-up	5	x	100		15
Set	2	x	200		30
	6	x	100	+	30
	2	x	200		10
	6	x	100	+	30
Cool-down	2	x	200		15

	Reps		Dist.	Inten.	Rest
Warm-up	4	x	150		15
Set	15	x	100		15
	15	x	50	+	10
Cool-down	5	x	100		20

	Reps		Dist.	Inten.	Rest
Warm-up	6	x	100		15
Set	1	x	200		25
	11	x	100		20
	11	x	50	+	15
	11	x	25	++	10
	1	x	200		25
Cool-down	2	x	300		15

LONG	Reps		Dist.	Inten.	Rest
Warm-up	8	x	50		15
Set	1	x	200	+	15
	3	x	400		25
	1	x	200	+	15
	3	x	400		25
Cool-down	5	x	100		15

	Reps		Dist.	Inten.	Rest
Warm-up	5	x	100		15
Set	4	x	300		10
	5	x	50	++	15
	4	x	300		20
Cool-down	4	x	150		15

	Reps		Dist.	Inten.	Rest
Warm-up	7	x	75		15
Set	5	x	500		60
Cool-down	6	x	100		15

Bike Workouts

Intervals	Reps		Time	Rest	Inten.	Spec.
Warm-up	1	x	15			
Set	10	x	2	2		
Cool-down	1	x	15			

Intervals	Reps		Time	Rest	Inten.	Spec.
Warm-up	1	x	15			
Set	5	x	2	1	+	Hard
	5	x	2	1		BGD
	5	x	1	1		SGD
Cool-down	1	x	15			

Intervals	Reps		Time	Rest	Inten.	Spec.
Warm-up	1	x	15			
Set	8	x	1	0		SLD
	5	x	1	1		BGD
	8	x	1	0		SLD
	5	x	1	1		SGD
	8	x	1	0		SLD
Cool-down	1	x	15			

Intervals	Reps		Time	Rest	Inten.	Spec.
Warm-up	1	x	15			
Set	6	x	5	3		
Cool-down	1	x	15			

Intervals	Reps		Time	Rest	Inten.	Spec.
Warm-up	1	x	15			
Set	10	x	1	1		BGD
	10	x	1	0	+	SGD
	20	x	0.5	0		SLD
Cool-down	1	x	15			

Intervals	Reps		Time	Rest	Inten.	Spec.
Warm-up	1	x	15			
Set	1	x	10	1		Hard
	20	x	1.5	0		SLD
	1	x	10	1	+	Hard
Cool-down	1	x	15			

Run Workouts

Intervals	Reps		Time	Rest	Inten.
Warm-up	1	x	15		
Set	4	x	1.5	1	
	3	x	4	2	
	2	x	8	3	
Cool-down	1	x	10		

Intervals	Reps		Time	Rest	Inten.
Warm-up	1	x	20		
Set	3	x	3	2	
	2	x	10	5	
	4	x	2	1	
Cool-down	1	x	15		

Intervals	Reps		Time	Rest	Inten.
Warm-up	1	x	15		
Set	8	x	3	2	
Cool-down	1	x	10		

Intervals	Reps		Time	Rest	Inten.
Warm-up	1	x	20		
Set	6	x	5	4	
Cool-down	1	x	15		

These workouts are just suggestions that can help you get to the finish line. You have to choose to use this tool to its fullest potential. To keep things fresh, try to select different speed workouts from week to week, and do your best to train in different areas from time to time. These workout charts will get you to the finish line, if that's what you decide you're going to do.

The Least You Need to Know

- Workout charts give you approximate time you should spend on each sport each day.

- Your heart rate zone during hard and speed workouts should be determined by the phase of training you're currently in.

- When selecting which interval workout to do, vary your selection from day to day or week to week.

- Choose interval workouts with longer intervals as you get closer to your race.

Chapter 15

Before and During Your Race

In This Chapter

- Nutrition and training as the race draws near
- Last-minute preparations
- Having a good mental approach to the race
- Staying at your pace

Okay, your race day is on the horizon. You've been training, and feel pretty good about the work you've put in. As your race approaches, it's important to keep a good head on your shoulders. Although it might be hard at times, try not to get too stressed out about physical, mental, or logistical factors. Your training schedule will help you reach your physical peak at the optimal time. Your mental preparation will have you in the right mind-set. As far as logistics go, you can verify last-minute details to reduce stress and unforeseen issues. You are going to do great!

Countdown to Race Day

Your training plan has this built into the schedule, but it is so important that we want to reiterate: you significantly cut back on the amount of time you spend working out as your race approaches. During the peak phase, the duration of your workouts decreases, but the intensity remains high initially. When the taper comes, you experience a mini-phase of considerably reduced activity just before your race. This part of your program can last between 10 and 21 days, depending on your current level of fitness and the race distance.

The programs in this book suggest starting the taper (at a minimum) the week before race week. The length of the taper should be longer for a greater-distance triathlon.

The longer the distance of your race, the more important this concept of staying off your feet becomes. If you're preparing for a super-sprint TRI, you might be out on the racecourse for 45 minutes or so. With a race of less than an hour, "extreme relaxing" during the week before your race might not have a serious impact on how you feel out on the course. If you're trying to conquer an Ironman, you could be out on the course for 17 hours. In that case, the more downtime you get in during your taper the better; your body will be that much more ready for a hard and long day.

Nutrition as the Time Draws Near

We've heard so many stories from people who followed a great training plan, tapered properly, had the best equipment, but then had terrible races. Why? They didn't keep up with their nutrition plan. In the days just before your race, stick with the nutrition that's worked for you throughout your training. Be wary of eating at restaurants, especially if you have a sensitive digestive system.

Nerves, psychological factors, or thirst might cause you to want to drink a lot of fluids. If that's the case, remember to drink a sports drink that contains electrolytes like sodium and potassium. If you drink excessive amounts of water (instead of sports drink), you'll dilute the amount of sodium and potassium in your system, which could lead to hyponatremia (discussed in further detail in Chapter 9). You might not feel it until you're in the thick of the race and you have a cramp that you just can't seem to shake. Hydrate in the days before your race, but be sure to include electrolytes!

Mentally Preparing for the Big Day

Mental preparation can be as important as physical preparation. If your mind isn't ready for the upcoming physical test, you could find yourself feeling unprepared and extremely anxious. But you've made it this far through your training, so you can relax, knowing you've put in good, quality training. Race day is a time to cash in on all that hard work. You'll be ready to go when the time comes.

Gravel Ahead

When doing any mental preparation for a race, don't only visualize a picturesque day with calm waters, no wind, and a flat racecourse. Preparing yourself for all the things that *might* go wrong will have you ready to face anything fate sends your way.

Don't sell mental preparation short. When you think about *visualization*, you might picture a bunch of yogis or monks chanting with their palms turned skyward. You can choose to meditate that way, or you can more systematically run through the events that will occur and make mental notes on those items you're not sure you're fully prepared for. Try to picture the different parts of your race, as well as the days and then minutes leading up to the start. When those moments come in real time, hopefully you'll be more comfortable because you've already "been through it" once before.

A relaxed mental state on race day helps you stay focused throughout the entire experience. If you're relaxed, you'll be able to think clearly and put all your concentration toward the task ahead of you. Practicing getting into this relaxed mental state several times in the weeks leading up to the race makes it that much easier for you.

You Can Do It!

The bottom line to this entire idea of mental preparation in the final weeks is that *you can do it!* Your body knows you can do it, because you've put in the time and effort. Logically, your mind knows it, too. However, doubt is a powerful adversary, and you might need to give it the beat-down.

You might have started the training program a week or two after you hoped. You might have to skip a training session here or there because of your job, or family, or passion for bonsai tree grooming. You might have pushed yourself too hard in one (or several) workout sessions. This has happened to everyone at some point or another. Life happens. People have to make choices and sacrifices, but as long as you were able to fit in most of the main workouts in your training program, you'll be prepared for your race. Have confidence in your preparation and in yourself, and go out there and do your best.

Check Your List, Check It Twice

Don't wait until the day before race day to make a list of all the things you want to verify and all the items you want to bring. On the next page is a sample race equipment checklist; you can use it as a base and adjust it as your experience throughout your season dictates. Some of the items are optional, and don't be afraid to add any additional items to the list. Utilize anything that's worked for you in training.

While you're checking things off your list, be sure to think about (and do more than think about if necessary) your travel plans. If you're traveling to another place for your race (meaning you have made any sort of travel arrangements), confirm your arrangements at least a week ahead of time. Check your:

- Flight reservations
- Airline rules about oversized luggage (bike)
- Car rental reservations (if applicable)—will the vehicle accommodate a bike/bike box?
- Hotel reservations
- Weather reports

Although in today's electronic world of immediate e-mail confirmations it's rare to have a lost reservation, the few minutes it takes to confirm can't hurt. Make a couple calls or e-mail inquiries, and solidify your peace of mind.

Race-Day Checklist

Swim	Run
❏ Swimsuit/trisuit	❏ Socks
❏ Wetsuit	❏ Shoes
❏ Wetsuit bag	❏ Shorts
❏ Lubrication	❏ Race outfit
❏ Swim cap (usually supplied)	❏ Race number
❏ Goggles	❏ Race belt
❏ Sunscreen	❏ Fuel belt
❏ Towel	❏ Hat
❏ Supplies to rinse feet after swim	❏ Sunglasses
❏ Defog	❏ Nutrition
❏ Earplugs and nose plugs	

Bike	Tri Bag/Other
❏ Bicycle	❏ Race checklist
❏ Helmet	❏ Photo ID/License
❏ Cycling shorts	❏ USAT membership card
❏ Jersey or singlet	❏ Race instructions
❏ Bike shoes	❏ Race maps
❏ Socks	❏ Timing chip
❏ Race number (bib)	❏ Eyeglasses/contacts
❏ Lubrication	❏ Flashlight
❏ Sunglasses	❏ Toilet paper
❏ Pump, CO_2, spare tube(s)	❏ Towel(s)
❏ Water bottles/energy drinks	❏ Duct tape or marker
❏ Bike multi-tool	❏ Chain lube
❏ Race belt	❏ Floor pump
❏ Race wheels	❏ Clothes (postrace)
❏ Nutrition	❏ First-aid kit
	❏ Nutrition
	❏ Heart-rate monitor
	❏ Fuel—sodium, etc.
	❏ Goggles—extra pair
	❏ MP3 player

> **Gravel Ahead** _____
>
> Don't wait until the last minute to schedule a prerace tune-up. Many other triathletes could be planning on getting their bike tweaked around the same time as you. Call ahead to the bike shop and get your tune-up done a little bit ahead of time to avoid the rush. If your tune-up falls only a day or two before your race, be sure you get out and go for a ride to verify your bike is in perfect working order.

Check-In and Packet Pickup

Race check-in usually occurs on the day before or the morning of a race. Some races offer both options, while other races offer only one. Many Ironman-distance races only offer check-in during certain hours 2 and 3 days before the race. Be sure you confirm the race check-in time and allow yourself enough time to take care of it. The lines at some of the larger races can twist and wind like those at an amusement park, so depending on your race, don't expect to get in and out quickly. Be prepared to wait a while, and do your best to show up at off times that might have shorter lines.

Oftentimes you'll receive a packet that includes several items such as the following:

♦ Swim cap, colored or numbered based on your wave

♦ Timing chip to electronically monitor when you cross various points (usually only larger races utilize this technology)

♦ Race bib to display your race number

♦ Sticker with race number for your helmet

♦ Race number to tag your bike

♦ Loads of advertisements for other races and possibly free samples of different fitness nutrition products

> **Gravel Ahead** _____
>
> It's awesome that some companies throw product samples in your race packet or goodie bag. But don't try any of these products until _after_ the race. Throughout your training, you've figured out what works for you; don't throw something new into the mix now.

Generally, the racecourse map will be available on the Internet several weeks or months before the race actually takes place. You might want to print it off early in your training and post it somewhere you can study it, especially if it's at all confusing or if you don't have a chance to go see it for yourself ahead of time. If you don't get a chance to study it until the few days before, still take a look and get an idea of the course you'll be on. The check-in is a perfect time to ask any questions you might have about the course.

In general, most TRIs follow a relatively standard set of rules. In the United States, USA Triathlon (USAT) is the governing body that dictates these rules. Even non-USAT-sanctioned races generally follow the same rules. Be sure you review the rules for your TRI, and ask questions of a race official when you're not sure about anything.

Training Tips _____

Race bibs are almost always made of a very strong material that doesn't tear and can withstand water and other punishment. An extra-stiff race bib might feel uncomfortable during a race and even cut you if your jersey rides up and the bib rubs directly on your skin. Before the race, crumple your race bib into a ball a few times to make it softer and less likely to cause you pain.

Good Morning, Race Day!

When race day comes, all the work you've been putting in will carry you through the day. You're ready for this!

To make this day go smoothly, treat it as if it were another training day. Approach it like you would any other day you planned on practicing all three sports. Sure, there are more people around than usual and there's that official starting line, but adopt the mind-set that it's just another day of training.

Be sure to wake up with enough time to eat, check and load up your gear, use the rest room, and get to the racecourse at least an hour before your race starts. If you want to get there even earlier to be safe, go for it.

At the Race

When you arrive at the venue, a buzz will fill the air. Take it all in, but don't let it get to you. It's okay to have butterflies in your stomach; just be sure they're flying in formation. Do not panic. Your goggles are going to keep the water out of your eyes. Your bike is going to perform just like it did in training. Your running shoes are fine. If you've adequately trained and followed the prerace checklist in this chapter, you're ready for this. Believe in yourself!

When you get to the race, your primary objectives are to check in (if you didn't check in a previous day), give your equipment a final check, and get *body marked*. Some people choose to kill two birds with one stone and ride their bike over to the body marking area. This way, you can confirm that your tires are properly inflated and get a chance to run through your gears. If you do this, wear your helmet!

def•i•ni•tion _____

Body marking is the act of having a race official or volunteer put your race number on your shoulder(s) and/or leg(s) using a marker or a stamp. Your sex and age might also be marked on some part of your body so your division is easily identifiable (for example, M35 would mean "male" and "35 years old").

Transition Setup

You should already have an idea about how to set up your transition area based on the transition workouts you did in training. But maybe you forgot something, so read this section!

For those of you completely new to the sport, the transition area looks like a bunch of elongated, metal construction horses. When you find the spot you want to claim, "double-check" (for the second time) that your bike tires are fully inflated and that you are in a very low (easy) gear. Lay claim to your territory by hooking your bike onto the horizontal rod in one of two ways:

♦ Hook the brakes of your handlebars over the rod.

♦ Slide your rear tire and seat under the rod and then lift the front end of the seat and place it on the rod.

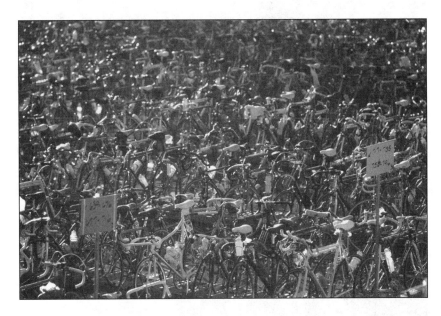

You may be assigned a specific row to set up your transition gear. If not, find the spot that feels right to you.

(Photo by Lois Schwartz)

Coaches' Corner

Be friendly and courteous in the transition area. Many people will be stressed before the start of the race, trying to remember if they got every piece of equipment and arranging all their gear. Striking up a conversation might help you (and others) forget about your nerves, and a friendly acquaintance is less likely to squeeze in on your already-tight real estate. Additionally, if you later realize that you forgot something such as sunscreen or a floor pump, a good neighbor might be more willing to share his or her supplies with someone who has been nice to them. Just like in any other aspect of life, a smile and a friendly attitude get you far.

When your bike is secured, be sure the water bottles you plan to ride with are filled and secure in their cages (if you're using some other sort of hydration system, be sure it's filled and ready). Then spread out your transition towel on the ground next to your bike so you can lay out your other equipment. Decide where you're going to put any discarded swim equipment after you're done with the first leg of the triathlon, and leave a space on the towel/ground for those things.

After practicing this during training, you should be familiar with the transition setup that works for you. It might look something like this.

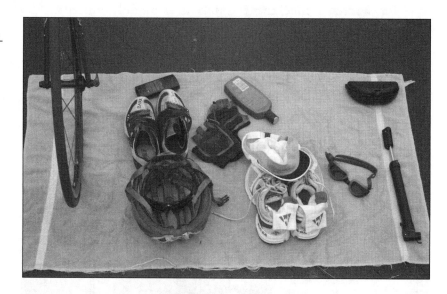

If you're wearing a wetsuit or trisuit in your race, be sure it's zipped all the way up and then head for the water.

(Photo by Lois Schwartz)

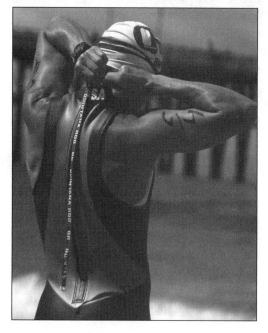

Last-Minute Preparations

Unless you're doing a half-Ironman distance or greater, you should warm up your muscles and get the blood flowing about 20 minutes before your race starts. The easiest way to do this is to go for a short jog (no more than 10 minutes) or swim a few strokes. If there's no time to warm up before the start of your race, don't worry about it. Just be sure you start at a reasonable pace when the race begins. For half-Ironman distance or longer (which could take between 4 and 17 hours), you don't want to waste any of your energy stores by warming up. When the race starts, take it slow and ease into your pace. That will serve as the perfect warm-up.

During the race, you're going to pass other triathletes, and other triathletes will pass you. You might be passed during the swim and then realize it's a little kid who looks like he should be in kindergarten. A granny on a bike right out of *The Wizard of Oz* might fly by you on the cycling portion of the race. Someone in the Clydesdale category (200 pounds or more) might run by you as you're approaching the finish line. Realize beforehand that this is going to happen, and when it does, just let it happen. Let it go. The beginning of your triathlon career is no time to let your ego talk you into going too hard. Do the best *you* can, and don't worry about anyone else.

Stay focused on the given moment. Don't get ahead of yourself and don't think about the next phase of the race. In the present you'll be most able to deal with a changing situation. Be prepared to pay attention to what's occurring around you. Focus on your intensity, know your nutrition plan, breathe, stay in the right rhythm, and make adjustments along the way.

> **Training Tips**
>
> Don't forget the lubes and creams. Pull your uniform back several inches in any spot where it covers your arms and legs and apply sunscreen in those spots. That way, if your jersey, shorts, or trisuit "rides up" during the race, your newly exposed skin will be protected.

On Your Mark, Get Set, Go!

Around 20 to 30 minutes prior to the start of the race, someone starts making announcements. Most race starts are separated into different *waves* (no pun intended). The order the different waves are called can vary. Usually, you'll know prior to the race based on race paperwork you received or the 411 on the event's website. In any case, listen for your wave to be called, and get to the swim start on time.

> **def•i•ni•tion**
>
> A **wave** is a group of triathletes based on age, sex, and sometimes weight (i.e., male Clydesdales who are 200+-pound athletes). For example, males 30 to 34 may all start together in a specific wave. Typically, each wave has a different color swim cap.

Let's Get Wet!

Swimming is almost always the shortest segment of the race, both in distance and in time. However, swimming can be the scariest part of the day for someone who isn't mentally prepared for what's about to transpire. Don't panic! You will be prepared.

The key is to find the spot in the water that fits you best, don't worry about getting bumped by other swimmers, and remember that it's okay to take a break if you need it.

The starting line may be in the water or on the beach. Wherever it is, find a spot in the crowd where you're comfortable.

(Photo by Lois Schwartz)

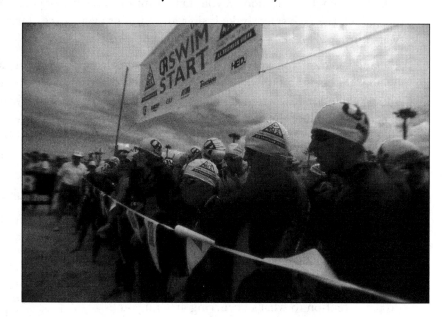

def•i•ni•tion

The **dolphin technique** is a way to avoid being pounded by large waves in the ocean or a lake. Simply dive beneath the large waves and come up after they've passed overhead. If you're in shallow-enough water that you touch the sea/lake floor, use that sand to push off to return to the surface.

The start of the triathlon follows one of two methods. Either everyone stands behind a line out of the water, or everyone is in the water behind a set of buoys or other makers. Either way, when the gun goes off, everyone heads for the most direct route to the first turn buoy. If you have to force your way through any large waves, try to use the *dolphin technique.*

Almost all triathlons start with the athletes in a pack with champion swimmers positioned in the front of the group. If you weren't the captain of your swim team or are new to triathlon, position yourself somewhere "comfortable." If you're an average swimmer and feel relatively confident being close to other people in the water, move to the middle of the crowd. If you have some reservations about being around a lot of people in the water or you know you're a slow swimmer, try placing yourself near the back and/or on the far side of the bunch. Basically, the closer to the front and "inside" you are, the less distance you have to swim. The farther to the back and "outside" you place yourself, the less stress you'll go through.

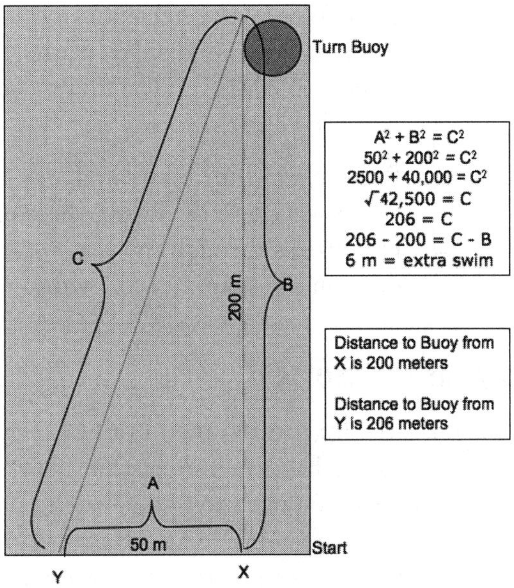
Turn Buoy
A² + B² = C²
50² + 200² = C²
2500 + 40,000 = C²
√42,500 = C
206 = C
206 - 200 = C - B
6 m = extra swim
C
200 m
B
Distance to Buoy from X is 200 meters
Distance to Buoy from Y is 206 meters
A
50 m
Start
Y
X

Geometry tells us that being at position Y adds some distance to the course, but we promise it's not much and it's worth it to feel comfortable. Check the math. A few meters are worth peace of mind!

Your first few strokes may be lacking in form. You might not be able to extend your reach completely because someone's feet are in your face. You might not be able to pull correctly because someone is snuggled up next to you. Don't panic! When the madness of the start subsides and you get into your groove, run through this mental checklist of the form items you've worked on:

- ❑ Chest down, butt up.
- ❑ Reach for it.
- ❑ Swim "on your side."

Training Tips

The swim primarily works your upper body. When you're getting to the final part of the swim, start kicking more forcefully. This brings more blood into your legs and helps prepare you for getting vertical in the next stage.

Sighting and Drafting

Competitive open-water swimming is more challenging not only because of the hordes of people, but also because this body of water doesn't have lane lines to guide you. Sometimes you can simply follow the crowd. However, this only works if the crowd is going straight. Therefore, it's good to incorporate sighting every few breaths by using other swimmers; a target buoy; or landmarks such as a building, lifeguard tower, or other large structure (as discussed in Chapter 5).

Gravel Ahead

Drafting is legal during the swim portion of the triathlon, but almost never legal during the bike! Be sure to remember when this is legal and illegal.

Hopefully, you've been able to practice sighting during your open-water workouts. No matter how you do it, do your best to stay on course. If you don't, you'll be adding extra distance to your race.

Remember, drafting behind another swimmer enables you to conserve energy during the race. Why? The front swimmer breaks through the water and reduces the amount of drag on the swimmer following.

Hope for the Best, Prepare for the Worst

The one thing that has the potential for causing the most heartache in the swim is the sudden feeling of claustrophobia. This has happened to triathletes of all levels, so don't be ashamed or let it make you think that you need to pull yourself out of the race if it happens to you. If you have the feeling that you're about to be struck with an anxiety attack, stop swimming, flip onto your back, and float or just tread water for a bit. Move to the outside of the pack if you can. If not, don't worry. Look up at the sky and think about how much space there really is for you. Take a few deep breaths and just relax. Tell yourself you are prepared and you can get through this. When you feel that you've calmed down enough, start swimming again. Don't worry about any lost time.

Swim starts can sometimes be a bit frantic, but stay calm and you'll be fine.

(Photo by Lois Schwartz)

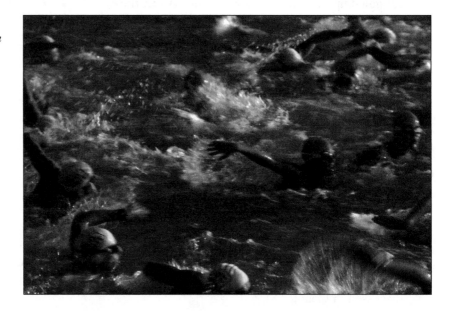

Swim to Bike: T1

Coming out of the water for your first transition (T1) is exciting. You're going from a state of sensory deprivation to one of sensory overload. You're going to be pumped up, but you need to keep two particular things in mind during T1:

- *Quadruple-check* that your helmet is on and latched.

- *Do not mount* your bike until you are out of the transition area and past the *mount/dismount line.*

Disobeying either of these rules will probably cost you some sort of penalty or disqualification, as they both have directly to do with the overall safety of the race.

def•i•ni•tion

The **mount/dismount line** is the boundary after which athletes can get on their bike coming out of T1 or before which they need to get off their bike going into T2. Do not violate this sacred line!

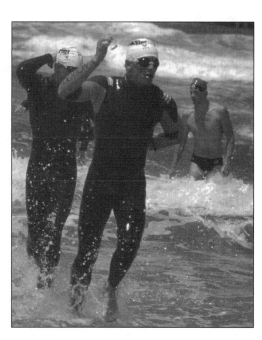

As soon as you head out of the water, start removing whatever gear you can while you're still on the move.

(Photo by Lois Schwartz)

On the Bike

Although a crowd is most likely cheering you on right out of transition, be sure you don't go out like a rocket! Start off slow. Gradually increase your intensity until you reach your race pace and RPM range of 80 to 100. Going out too hard causes lactic acid to begin to flow, so stay aerobic. This is especially important for Ironman and half-Ironman athletes. Becoming anaerobic requires a period of metabolic recovery, which reduces efficiency and quickly depletes glycogen stores. Especially in the longer races, you don't want to fade during the final miles of the bike course. Proper pacing is the key.

Make yourself comfortable and find your groove. Depending on the race distance, you might have hours ahead. Have patience and enjoy the ride.

Training Tips

Feel your pedal stroke. Remember to imagine spinning in small circles. Focus on the pull at the bottom of the stroke, and recruit those hamstrings and glutes.

Proper gearing is the key to maintaining pace and keeping maximum efficiency. Remember what you learned in training and shift as often as necessary. Gearing is individual to each triathlete's abilities, as well as to the topography of each racecourse. Remember that this is your race. Don't try to mirror other athletes' gearing choices. Find *your* gear.

When riding in a line, be sure to leave three bike lengths between yourself and the next biker to avoid a drafting penalty.

(Photo by Lois Schwartz)

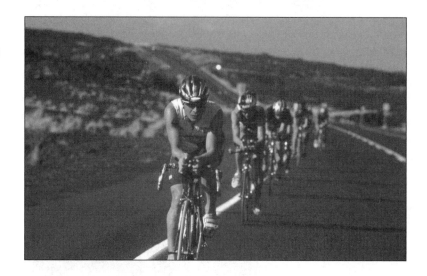

Gravel Ahead

During the ride, you might come across a race marshal. The marshals are there to guide you, warn you of traffic, and enforce such violations as drafting. Although race marshals have authority over the race participants, they do not have the authority to stop vehicular traffic. Some courses are closed to cars; some are not. Always be vigilant, especially when crossing intersections. Marshals are usually not trained professionals; they are fellow triathletes or friends volunteering their time. Show them respect, and if you have breath to spare, a "thank you" is always welcome.

"Soft hands" and a little give in your arm will help in the aid-station hand-offs.

(Photo by Lois Schwartz)

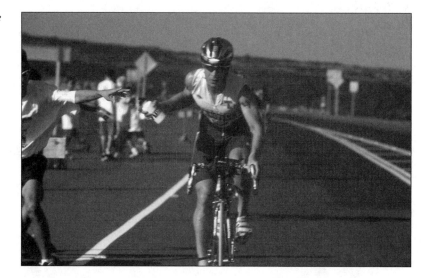

Settle In and Chill

After a few miles in the saddle, your muscles might feel tight, so it's a good idea to mix up the ride to stretch out your body. Stand up from time to time and give your back a break. You can also sit tall and roll your neck and head. While stretching, be sure to keep your eyes on the road and stay in control of your bike. In addition to these strategies, remember our tips from the bike chapter: ride with a quiet upper body and loose fingers. Stay relaxed and conserve energy. Activate only the muscles needed.

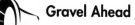

Gravel Ahead

Avoid temperature-related illness such as heat stroke. If the temperature or humidity is significantly higher than you expected, you'll need to exceed your planned fluid and electrolyte intake.

If your race is long enough to warrant fueling up, the bike segment is the best time to consume most of your calories. However, keep in mind that many triathletes need to allow their stomachs time to settle after a swim before eating. Therefore, as a rule of thumb, "gradual is good."

Bike to Run: T2

You'll have a sense of accomplishment and relief as you dismount the bike in the marked zone to enter the second and final transition (T2). If your bike shoes are not rubber soled, be careful of your footing as you run into T2. Take your time and walk if you have to; a few seconds more in transition won't seriously impact your time.

Find your equipment, rack your bike, swap out your bike gear with your running stuff, and head back out on the course!

On the Run

The first mile on the run course typically feels awkward. Be patient and let your legs switch from bike mode to run mode. Your training transition runs will show their value here.

Watch your pace, especially at the beginning. Don't allow the crowds and adrenaline to push you faster than your intended speed. The goal on the run is to get from point A to point B in a smooth, balanced, relaxed fashion, and to get there efficiently. Aim for comfort and remember good form. Focus so that your energy is channeled to contribute to forward movement, and keep your shoulders, jaw, and arms relaxed.

Remember and repeat these running concepts in your head:

- ◆ Stand tall.

- ◆ Just breathe.

- ◆ Don't bounce.

- ◆ Keep a quicker cadence.

- ◆ Run relaxed.

- ◆ Land on your forefoot.

Staying hydrated during a longer race needs to be one of your top priorities. If necessary, go double fisted like Ironman legend Paula Newby-Fraser.

(Photo by Lois Schwartz)

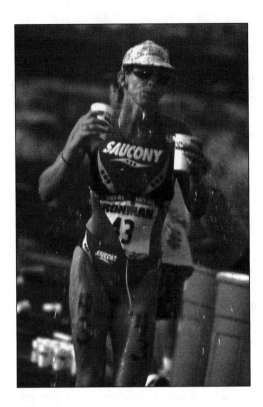

Woo! The Finish Line

As you approach the finish, you'll notice the cheer of the crowd increasing. Have fun with it. There's no rush to cross the line. It's your time to give high fives, jump up and down, or do a cartwheel if you want. Relish in the moment. Once you cross the line, you become an official triathlete!

The joy of finishing is a function of invested effort. Goals obtained through intense and focused effort are always the sweetest. That's why TRI is so addicting. Take it all in and then go celebrate with your fellow athletes and supporters.

Past the Finish Line

After you've had a moment to enjoy your huge accomplishment, be sure you take some time to refuel and cool down. Most races offer some sort of food and drink to athletes near the finish line. Even if you don't feel thirsty, be sure to get a lot of fluids to replenish what you lost.

Keep walking or otherwise moving. You want to let your body manage itself (heart rate, stress hormones, lactic acid levels, etc.) before you just stop moving abruptly. Take a few minutes to go through some or all of the stretches discussed in Chapter 10. Your body will thank you later.

Once you're cooled down and you've had some refueling time, head back to the transition area to pick up your belongings. You may be asked to show your race bib to enter the transition area (to keep nonathletes out). Additionally, you might not be able to reenter the transition area if some athletes have not yet completed T2. Once you do enter transition, double-check that you pick up all your gear as well as any trash that might be yours.

While collecting your gear, try to make a mental note of the organization that worked in transition and the things you could do better next time. There will be a next time ... right?

The Least You Need to Know

- Don't make any drastic changes to your training or nutrition regiment in the days leading up to the race.

- Know the schedule of events, and be sure to give yourself enough time so you don't have to rush.

- Treat the TRI race like a training day, and keep self-monitoring your form.

- Swim, bike, and run at *your* pace, and don't worry about what any other athletes are doing.

- Be sure to enjoy every minute of your TRI experience.

Chapter 16

That Was *Awesome!* What's Next?

In This Chapter

- ◆ Evaluating your race performance
- ◆ Planning your next TRI adventure
- ◆ What to do in the off-season or in your "retirement"
- ◆ Applying TRI to life

You've completed your first triathlon. Congratulations! Now let's take a step back and regroup. How did things go? What did you think? It's good to document the experience with notes and impressions and then build on it.

Did the TRI bug bite you? Can you feel this amazing sport coursing through your veins? Almost every person who crosses the starting line as a triathlete wants it to happen again and again. If this feeling didn't happen to you, don't worry about it. Let's still evaluate your big day, and maybe you can revisit your desires again at a later date.

Recapture That Feeling

Crossing the finish line in a triathlon, especially one that created a real personal challenge to prepare for, is a feeling like nothing else. Maybe you had a pain in your side and that "feeling like nothing else" was not completely positive. Perhaps something happened and you weren't able to finish the race at all.

No matter what happened, we're willing to bet you experienced intense feelings of joy at some point during your day. Maybe they struck you when you were coming down the home stretch toward the finish line. Maybe it was when you were about to complete the swimming or biking leg. Maybe it was even earlier, like when the race started. Do you remember the last time you felt like that?

How Did You Do?

When you're ready to give yourself some constructive criticism, find a comfortable position in a familiar spot. Have a notebook or a laptop handy so you can take a note or two. Ask yourself:

♦ Did you arrive at the race venue with enough time to check in, get body marked, set up your transition area, etc.?

♦ Did you get to the starting line too early, too late, or just right?

♦ How did you feel during each leg of the triathlon?

♦ How was your pace?

♦ How was your nutrition strategy?

♦ How did you feel right at the end of your race?

♦ When you crossed that line, did you feel like you gave it everything you had? Or that you could have kept on going?

♦ What could you have done differently?

Probe your memory and try to get a real picture of how you feel you did, regardless of your time.

Needless to say, most everyone who races has a "lesson learned" at the end of a race (and probably several). Don't let that bother you at all, because learning lessons is what this sport is all about. We are constantly trying to improve ourselves so our next attempt will be even more successful. Even the most elite athletes are constantly learning and bettering themselves with regards to training, nutrition, pace, and recovery.

Plan Your Next Adventure

Perhaps you completed your TRI and you feel like you accomplished everything you set out to do. Maybe you want to call it a season, or perhaps call it a career. If that's your choice, we support you all the way! However, we're guessing that the TRI bug will bite many of you. You might feel the need to keep setting TRI-oriented goals in your life. If the race season isn't over, maybe you'll choose to conquer another TRI. If the season is over, maybe you'll pick out one or a few races you'd like to do the following year.

A new-distance race is definitely an attainable goal. If the TRI season isn't over after your original goal race, you might consider doing another one this year. If you can get to one that's at least a couple weeks away and still accepting entries, you could think about signing up. If you've trained specifically for a certain distance TRI, you don't want to sign up for a longer race if there's little time to prepare or recover between events. A race of the same distance or shorter would probably be your safest bet. If you do have some time before that next race and you want to increase your training duration, a longer race might be in order.

> **Coaches' Corner**
>
> Maybe you want to focus on the off-season instead. What sort of goals do you want to accomplish while you're not racing? Maybe you want to get stronger through lifting, thinner by dieting and training, or stronger at one of the three sports. Whichever you decide to do, we suggest writing down your goals and posting them somewhere you'll see them on a regular basis.

If the season is coming to a close shortly after you complete your goal race, you'll have to set your sights on next year's race schedule. Unless you're signing up for a very popular race, like an Iron-man, you probably don't have to commit to a specific race an entire season in advance. However, you can still spend some time thinking about what sort of goals you'd like to have for next year:

- How did training go this season?

- Did you feel like the amount of training you did fit in well with your lifestyle?

- Did you often feel like training was taking up too much of your time or was too difficult?

- Was it extremely easy? Do you wish you had more volume and intensity?

- Will your lifestyle remain the same during the next season, or will any factors reduce (marriage, children, promotion) or increase (kids off to college, retirement) the amount of time you have to dedicate to training?

Your answers to those questions will help you gauge the race distance you'll have time to train for. Don't bite off more than you can chew. Keep it fun and enjoy the journey.

Get Involved

If you're totally comfortable where you are as far as racing goes but you want to expand your involvement in other ways, TRI provides ample opportunities for that. Several clubs and other organizations across the country offer people the ability to get involved. Ask a TRI friend, a race official, or check out Appendix B for some sites that will help get you started.

Join a TRI Club

Maybe you did this first one on your own because you weren't too sure how it was going to turn out, or even if you were going to complete it. Now that you have done it, you might feel a little more comfortable getting more social. If you're not already part of a TRI club, why don't you revisit that possibility now?

> **Coaches' Corner**
>
> A TRI club is not made up of a bunch of elite triathletes. A club is comprised of a bunch of athletes of varying goals, abilities, and ages. You absolutely will fit in with a TRI club.

Not only can workouts be more fun when you do them with a wide variety of personalities, but you also have opportunities to pick up countless (and sometimes priceless) tips from the members who have more experience than you do. Clubs are also a great way to create an athletic network, which can be helpful in finding races, carpooling to them, and having a fun time socializing afterward. We encourage you to consider a TRI club if you haven't already.

Volunteer for an Event

Volunteering is a great way to give back. Before you did your first TRI, you probably didn't think that the volunteers really affected the racers too much. After your first, you probably realized that without volunteers, organized TRI events would not be possible.

> **Coaches' Corner**
>
> Even while you're training for a TRI, you can still volunteer your time at another event. Being a volunteer lets you watch all the different athletes from all across the spectrum of ability. Watching the race as an outsider might give you that extra spark of inspiration you're looking for. Not to mention you'll gain a stronger sense of appreciation for what volunteers bring to the event.

Off-Season Dining

When you finish your big race or complete your training for the season, your body will probably go through some changes. During the season, your activity levels are increased, and so is your caloric intake. When the season ends or you back off the intensity of your training, you should also back off your caloric intake. If you don't, you'll start putting on some unwanted pounds. It makes perfect sense, but sometimes people forget to stop and think about it.

The important thing to keep in mind is that you don't *need* to eat as many calories in the off-season as you were during the season. Most likely, you got into a habit of dining and consuming a relatively standard amount of calories each day while you were working out hard. In the off-season, you need to break your eating pattern and reevaluate how much food you really need to take in on a daily basis. To maintain a desired weight, remember: *calories ingested should equal calories burned.*

There are some good free calorie calculators available online. You input some specifics such as body weight, age, gender, and some general-to-specific daily activities, and the magic of the Internet estimates your daily requirements. This gives you a pretty good idea of how many calories are required to meet energy demands (see Appendix B).

Gravel Ahead

Don't think you can continue to eat whatever you want because you're a triathlete (unless you're keeping your training relatively consistent and intense, that is). Be smart, because it'll be a pain to have to lose those few extra pounds at the beginning of the next season.

Applying Triathlon in Life

You've probably already realized this, but TRI serves as a great metaphor for life: any goal is attainable; all you need is desire, hard work, and perseverance; if you put your mind to it … well, you get the drift. The point is that TRI is not easy, but "average" people become triathletes all the time. Why? Because they believe.

If you want to achieve something in life, you can use the same process you did in TRI:

1. Decide on a goal.

2. Evaluate how much time and resources you can dedicate to that goal.

3. Lay out a plan to get to where you need to be.

4. Start executing your plan.

5. Deal with any potholes you encounter along the way.

6. Achieve your goal and then think, *What's next?*

TRI teaches this priceless gift: live in the now. *How's my stroke … how's my pace … how's my stride …?* TRI forces you to focus on what's happening *right now*. It's important to always be in the moment, both in TRI and in life. For example, you can quit worrying by simply acknowledging the now. Most worries, fears, and any other negatives exist in our thoughts of the past or future. Stay present. Listen to your breathing, feel your heart beat, smell the air ….

As you employ your senses, you'll find it heightens the power of now. When your attention shifts from a future outcome to the present action, TRI and life flow naturally.

Triathlon is much more than swimming, biking, and running. It can be a way of life, a philosophy, a lifestyle. Be in the moment. Stay fit. Challenge yourself. Evolve. Be flexible (literally and figuratively). Strive for a new PB (personal best). Have fun. Don't take it too seriously. Wake early and seize the day. Find camaraderie. Hit the beach. Volunteer your time. Explore your surroundings. Shed a few unwanted pounds. Shave those legs. Manage your time better. Be strong.

The list goes on and on. We tried to touch on each dimension of this unique sport; we trust you'll discover some of that brilliance. We hope you all get involved and enjoy the journey.

Head off into the direction of your dreams.

(Photo by Lois Schwartz)

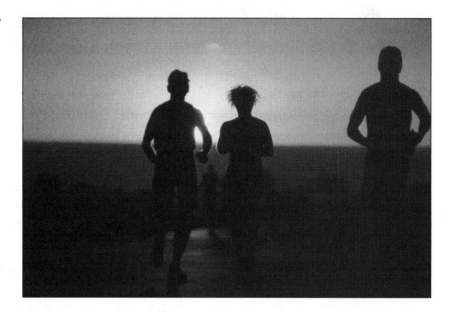

The Least You Need to Know

◆ Giving yourself constructive criticism on pace, nutrition, transitions, and equipment helps you better prepare for your next event.

◆ One TRI down—now what? Now's the time to start planning for another race or decide how you can stay involved with TRI.

◆ The lessons of TRI can be applied to life; approaching life with a TRI mind-set can improve both your life's quality and enjoyment.

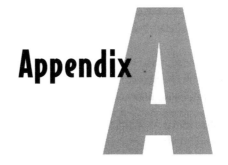

Glossary of Common TRI Terms

acceleration   Increase of running speed over a fixed distance; starting with a slow jog and ending almost at a sprint.

active recovery   Using exercise at lower levels of intensity to promote recovery.

aero bars   A combination of handlebars and elbow supports on your bike that enables you to get your head and shoulders lower and more forward than you would be able to with regular handlebars. This position improves your overall aerodynamics and decreases stress on your back.

aerobic system   Aerobic means "with oxygen"; aerobic system is a method of internal energy production that occurs when oxygen is present.

age groupers   All nonprofessional triathlon competitors.

aid stations   Volunteers set up at specific points throughout a race who offer athletes hydration/nutrition options (as well as moral support).

American valve   *See* shrader valve.

anaerobic threshold   *See* lactate threshold (LT).

arm warmers   Polyester material worn tightly from your wrist to your upper arm (in conjunction with a short-sleeve or sleeveless jersey), used to keep you warm during cooler conditions. They can be pulled off easily and stored in a bike jersey pocket when you warm up.

ATP (adenosine triphosphate)   An energy phosphate molecule required to provide energy production for cellular function. It can be produced both aerobically and anaerobically.

ballistic stretching   Semi-rapid uncontrolled stretching movements like bouncing. The purpose of this type of stretching is to mimic activities that are dynamic in nature, but this is a higher-risk technique and most experts do not advocate it for the general population.

base phase   The first layer of the training pyramid. During the base phase we develop endurance and strength that carry the weight of future "layers." In this phase, you're still honing and developing skills, and most workouts are in heart rate zones 1 and 2.

Bento box   A nylon box that sits on the top tube of your bicycle, behind the stem. It provides storage of things such as nutrition gels or bars.

bike box   A hard case used to pack a disassembled bike for easy transport or storage.

bike computer   A tiny computer mounted on a bike, used to monitor data such as speed, distance, time, pedal rotations per minute, elevation change, etc.

bilateral breathing   Alternating breaths between your left and right sides during swimming.

bonk   A slang term used to describe the act of running out of energy before the race is over. This can happen from pushing too hard, improper fueling, or a combination of both.

build   To increase speed throughout a swim.

build phase   The second layer of the training pyramid in which workouts increase in intensity and duration. Heart rate should hover primarily between zones 2 and 3.

bursitis   Inflammation or irritation of the bursa (small fluid-filled sacs between joints).

cadence   The measure or beat of a specific movement (breathing, heart beat, pedaling, etc.). In cycling terminology, cadence refers to pedal revolutions per minute (RPM).

caffeine   A natural stimulant used in many types of sport energy supplements.

calorie   A unit of energy supplied by food and released upon oxidation by the body.

cardiac output (Q)   The amount of blood pumped from the left ventricle during one heart beat.

chain ring   The front gearing of a bike. It's made of metal teeth that the chain sits on.

chondromalacia patella (runner's knee)   An irritation of the undersurface of the kneecap (patella). In certain individuals or stemming from overuse, the kneecap rubs against one side of the knee joint and the cartilage surface become irritated, resulting in knee pain.

clincher tire   A tire that "clinches" to the rim of a wheel. It tucks into the rim and is secured by the air pressure from the inner tube. This is the standard tire that is found on most recreational bicycles.

clipless pedals   Pedals that lock to the cleat of a bike shoe (like a ski binding). Pedals of this type enable cyclists to generate maximum power in every rotation.

CO_2 cartridge   A small cylinder of compressed CO_2 that can be released through a regulator valve (adaptor) to inflate a tire.

creatine phosphate system   An anaerobic system within the body that kicks in at high intensities. It is suitable for single or continuous short bursts of energy lasting a few seconds.

cross-training   To attain fitness through more than one type of exercise.

descend   To complete several intervals of the same distance, with a decrease in time with each set.

dolphin technique   Diving beneath large waves and coming up after they've passed overhead while swimming out to sea.

drafting   To move close behind a moving object so as to take advantage of the slipstream (water or air). Drafting is illegal during the bike portion in almost all TRI races.

economy   The efficiency in which an activity is performed. How efficiently your body works to get you from point A to point B is your economy.

electrolytes   Nutrients required by cells to internally regulate hydration (sodium, potassium, etc.).

endorphins   Peptide hormones released during exercise that reduce the sensation of pain and increase the feelings of joy.

ergogenic aids   Anything that improves (or is thought to improve) one's performance. *Ergo* = "work"; *genic* = "gives rise to."

European valve   *See* presta valve.

fartlek   Swedish for "speed play," a fartlek involves a warm-up and then a series of shorter, up-paced periods defined by distance between landmarks (city blocks), time, or general feel.

fatigue   The decreased capacity to function normally because of excessive stimulation or prolonged exertion.

fins   Swimming shoes that increase the surface area of the feet and enable the user to generate more power with each kick.

flexibility   The range of motion within a joint.

frequency   The number of workouts performed in a given time frame.

glucosamine   A supplement associated with improved joint function.

glutamine   A supplement that's been associated with improved capacity for recovery because of its ability to improve glucose absorption. It's a naturally occurring substance in the body.

glycogen   The stored form of glucose.

hand paddles   Plastic paddles that strap to a swimmer's hands and enable the swimmer to generate more power with each stroke.

hardware   Any award won in a triathlon, such as medals or trophies, usually given out to the top finishers per age group.

heart rate monitor   A combination chest strap and watch receiver. The monitor detects the heart rate and sends a signal to the watch receiver, which displays the heart rate.

heat stroke   An extremely dangerous condition that occurs when the body can no longer cool itself, resulting from prolonged exposure to excessive heat. Symptoms include absence of sweat, severe headache, high fever, hot dry skin, and, in serious cases, collapse and coma.

heel spur   A growth of bone that occurs when the body tries to heal itself after a severe tear in the plantar fascia.

hydration system   Any method an athlete uses to carry hydration fluids during activity, such as water bottles or backpack bladders.

hydrodynamics   The study of the efficiency of an object moving through water (or any other liquid).

hydrotherapy   External use of water in the medical treatment of certain ailments.

hyponatremia   Low blood sodium levels.

iliotibial (IT) band syndrome   Excessive friction caused between the IT band (a large tendon that runs along the outside of the leg from the knee to the hip) and the knee or hip bone, often caused by improper running or biking technique. The result is typically a sharp pain on either side of the knee but can also cause pain in the hip region.

indoor bike trainer   A device that allows any standard bicycle to become a stationary workout machine, with varying levels of resistance.

intensity   The stress level placed on the body.

interval   To work out with several periods of high intensity and a designated period of recovery. The periods are marked by distance or time.

kick board   A lightweight, foam board used to help keep the upper body afloat during swimming.

lace locks   Small plastic devices used in conjunction with existing laces to tighten or loosen shoes quickly and efficiently.

lactate (lactic acid)   A waste product of the anaerobic system known to cause muscle fatigue.

lactate threshold (LT)   The level of exercise intensity whereby lactate begins to rapidly accumulate in the blood faster than it can be metabolized.

large gear drills (LGD)   A cycling drill performed using both legs in a large gear and a low RPM; great for increasing muscular strength and endurance.

mantra   A word or phrase repeated over and over to increase focus and motivation.

master's swim workout   An organized and coached workout with specific goals.

minerals   Naturally occurring, inorganic elements. In this book, only minerals that are nutrients are discussed.

mitochondria   Subcellular structures that help metabolize units of food into energy.

mount/dismount line   The boundary during a triathlon after which athletes can get onto their bike coming out of T1 or before which they need to get off their bike going into T2.

neutral   While running, to strike and then roll through the middle of the foot and off the middle or front section of the foot.

never-ending pool   A swimming apparatus that allows for stationary swimming with the use of a constant flow of water current.

organic   Anything that derives from a living organism.

orthotics   A term used to describe custom-made shoe inserts that correct slight abnormalities in joints.

osteoporosis   A disease in which the bones become extremely porous, are subject to fracture, and heal slowly. Post-menopausal women are at increased risk for this disease.

overload   To push one's body to levels beyond a certain threshold (but below tolerance levels), to force beneficial adaptations that will occur in response to those demands.

overtraining   An advanced stage of fatigue caused from training beyond your body's ability to cope.

pace   The rate of speed at which an activity or movement proceeds.

PAR-Q (physical activity readiness questionnaire)   A basic screening form used to decide if a person is ready for a certain type of physical activity.

peak phase   The final layer of the training pyramid in which the training duration begins to decrease, frequency remains constant, and intensity increases. Intensity should be maintained primarily in zones 3 and 4 during key workouts, while other workouts should be done at low intensity—zones 1 and 2.

periodization   The blending of workloads, progression, and recovery such that optimal gains in fitness can occur at optimal times.

plantar fasciitis   Inflammation in the heel region of the foot characterized by pain during activity, such as walking or running.

preparation phase   The foundation upon which the training pyramid is built. Fitness demands are introduced and technique is improved. The heart rate should remain primarily in zone 1.

presta valve   A long and thin wheel air valve, usually used for road bikes.

progression   A strategy of gradually increasing workload to maximize fitness benefits.

pronation   While running, to strike, roll inward and forward, and then push off the ball of the foot or big toe.

proprioceptive neuromuscular facilitation (PNF)   A type of stretching that involves a contract-relax sequence.

pull buoy   A foam device that can be squeezed between the legs during swimming to help lift the lower body.

purse   In triathlon, the monetary prize for winning.

race wheels   Nonstandard bicycle wheels used to improve aerodynamics.

rate of perceived exertion (RPE)   A scale developed by Dr. Gunnar Borg to measure one's subjective (based on feel) intensity.

repeats   A repetition of a specific distance or time within an interval.

rest   Recovery time taken after a period of increased effort, such as an interval.

reversibility   The decline of the body's fitness level after discontinuing a training program.

seat pack (saddlebag)   A general storage pouch hanging from a saddle or over the rear wheel of a bicycle.

set   A series of two or more repetitions of increased effort over a given distance or time.

shin splints   Pains along the tibia or shinbone of the lower leg. The pain runs vertically along the inside or outside of the bone and is often caused from adding too much exercise volume too fast as well as general overuse.

shrader valve   Short and thick wheel air valve (like those on a car).

sighting   Using distant landmarks to keep on course while swimming in open water.

single leg drills (SLD)   Cycling drills performed one leg at a time (with clipless pedals), in which only one leg is used to rotate the pedals at a time; great for developing and improving the "full circle" mentality.

small gear drills (SGD)   Cycling drills performed using both legs with the chain in a very easy gear and high RPMs; help develop neuromuscular system by teaching it to fire efficiently at higher rates.

sodium   A critical electrolyte in the human body, especially with regards to hydration. Sodium replacement is extremely important during any long or hot workouts or races.

specificity   To generate a specific response by placing a specific demand on the body (e.g., cycling often makes an athlete's cycling muscles stronger).

Spinning   A group cycling class in which participants are instructed to vary their speed, resistance, and intensity throughout the workout.

static stretching   The preferred and most widely accepted method of stretching, which utilizes slow, gradual movements at low intensity.

stroke volume   The amount of blood pumped from each ventricle each time the heart beats.

supination   When a foot strikes the ground, rolls outward toward the outside of the foot, and then off the front-middle area of the foot/toes.

swimmer's shoulder   A condition characterized by soreness and inflammation of the rotator cuff muscle. It's most often caused by the freestyle stroke's repetitive overhead arm motion.

swimming velocity (SV) calculation   The distance traveled with each stroke (stroke length or SL) multiplied by the duration of each stroke (stroke rate or SR) or $SV = (SL) \times (SR)$.

taper   Reduction of frequency, intensity, and duration to allow maximum rest and readiness in the final days before a race.

target heart rate (THR)   The goal heart rate of a person participating in a fitness activity. $(THR) = (220 - Age) \times Desired\ Intensity\ \%$.

tempo   The speed at which a movement/exercise is conducted.

tempo run   A faster-than-normal pace, sustained for the designated period of time.

tendonitis   Inflammation of a tendon (band of fibrous tissue that connects muscle to bone) generally caused by overuse.

toe clips   Plastic clips attached to the forward side of a pedal or pedal straps that help secure your feet to a pedal while cycling.

transition area   The area designated for changing clothing and gear when going from one sport to another in a triathlon race.

transition runs (T-runs)   A training run performed within minutes of the completion of a training ride. This helps prepare a triathlete's body for an actual race.

TRI-bag   A backpack with specific compartments to organize TRI gear—shoes, helmet, wetsuit, etc.

tubular tire   One piece (tire and tube) that is wrapped around the wheel frame and inflated. Special wheel glue must be used to adhere the tire to the wheel.

vitamins   Organic compounds that are vital to life.

VO$_2$ max   The volume (in milliliters) of oxygen used per kilogram of body weight per minute (ml/kg/min).

wetsuit   A tight-fitting permeable suit worn in cold water to retain body heat.

Zen   A philosophy that relies heavily on obtaining enlightenment by way of meditation.

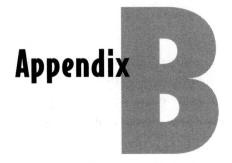

Appendix B

Resources

Throughout this book, we've given you a *ton* of information. If you still want more, you've turned to the right place. The resources in this appendix enable you to find more history and current events, delve deeper into specific techniques, and continue to learn about triathlon almost indefinitely.

Organizations

USA Triathlon (USAT)
www.usatriathlon.com
USAT is the national governing body for the multisport disciplines of triathlon, duathlon, aquathlon, and winter triathlon in the United States. It coordinates and sanctions thousands of multisport events across the country and works to create interest and participation in those programs. Membership in USAT is required for participation in USAT-sanctioned events. (One-day memberships are available for about one-forth the price of annual membership.)

Ironman Series
www.ironmanlive.com
World Triathlon Corporation (WTC) owns and organizes Ironman Triathlons across the world. It has recently added the Ironman 70.3 Series, bringing the Ironman total events to 40. The website provides information on events and offers live streaming video of some races to your PC.

Triathlon.org
www.triathlon.org
Triathon.org is the official site of the International Triathlon Union (ITU), the world governing organization for the sport of triathlon and the only triathlon body recognized by the International Olympic Committee.

USA Swimming
www.usaswimming.org
USA Swimming is the national governing body for the sport of swimming.

USA Cycling
www.usacycling.org
USA Cycling is a family of organizations that promote and govern different disciplines of the sport and work as one to build the sport of bicycle racing, assist with athlete development, and sustain international competitive excellence.

USA Track and Field
www.usatf.org
USA Track and Field (USATF) is the national governing body for track and field, long-distance running, and race walking in the United States.

American Dietetic Association (ADA)
www.eatright.org
The ADA is the nation's largest organization of food and nutrition professionals. ADA serves the public by promoting optimal nutrition, health, and well-being. ADA members are the nation's food and nutrition experts, translating the science of nutrition into practical solutions for healthy living.

Online Resources

You can find nearly anything online these days, including information on TRI. Here's just a sampling to get you started. Poke around, and you'll find many others.

TRI Beginners

www.beginnertriathlete.com   www.trinewbies.com

Locate and Sign Up

www.active.com   www.usms.org/placswim

www.trifind.com

General TRI

www.insidetri.com   www.trifuel.com

www.slowtwitch.com   www.xtri.com

www.transitiontimes.com

Magazines

www.competitor.com

www.triathletemag.com

www.runnersworld.com

Coaching

www.multisports.com

www.markallenonline.com

www.davescottinc.com

Just for the Ladies

www.hersports.com

www.irongirl.com

www.trichic.com

Other

www.nasports.com (previously
www.ironmannorthamerica.com)

www.runnersweb.com

www.velonews.com

www.gmap-pedometer.com

www.caloriecontrol.org
www.shipbikes.com

www.tribiketransport.com

www.teamintraining.org

www.triguys.net
www.stevekatai.com

Index

CHECK OUT THESE BEST-SELLERS

More than 450 titles available at booksellers and online retailers everywhere!

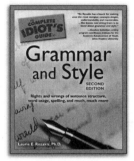

978-1-59257-115-4

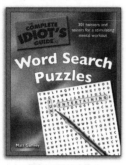

978-1-59257-900-6

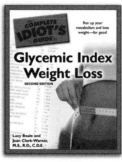

978-1-59257-855-9

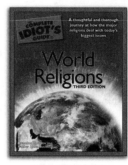

978-1-59257-222-9

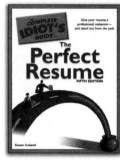

978-1-59257-957-0

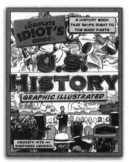

978-1-59257-785-9

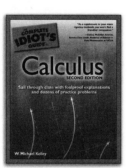

978-1-59257-471-1

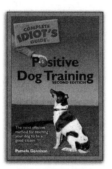

978-1-59257-483-4

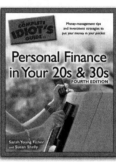

978-1-59257-883-2

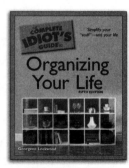

978-1-59257-966-2

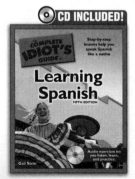

978-1-59257-908-2

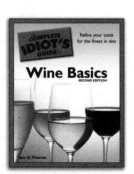

978-1-59257-786-6

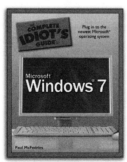

978-1-59257-954-9

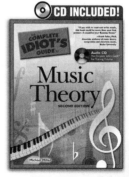

978-1-59257-437-7

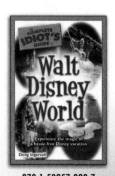

978-1-59257-888-7

ALPHA idiotsguides.com